Hearing and Aging

Ray H. Hull

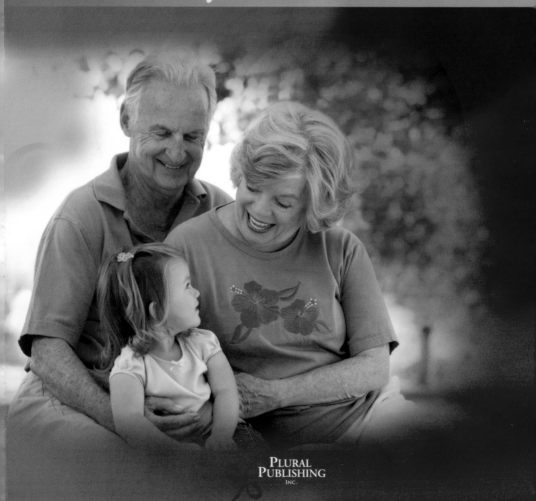

PLURAL
PUBLISHING
INC.

Hearing and Aging

Hearing and Aging

Ray H. Hull, PhD, FASHA, FAAA
Professor of Communication Sciences and Disorders,
Audiology/Neurosciences
Department of Communication Sciences and Disorders
College of Health Professions
Wichita State University
Wichita, Kansas

With information on Hearing Loss in Older Adulthood (Chapter 1) by
Gabrielle Saunders, PhD, and Dawn Konrad-Martin, PhD
National Center for Rehabilitative Auditory Research
Portland, Oregon

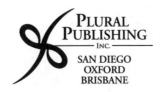

PLURAL
PUBLISHING
INC.
SAN DIEGO
OXFORD
BRISBANE

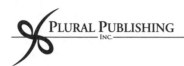

5521 Ruffin Road
San Diego, CA 92123

e-mail: info@pluralpublishing.com
Web site: http://www.pluralpublishing.com

49 Bath Street
Abingdon, Oxfordshire OX14 1EA
United Kingdom

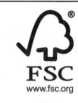

FSC
www.fsc.org
MIX
Paper from
responsible sources
FSC® C011935

Typeset in 11/14 Garamond by Flanagan's Publishing Services, Inc.
Printed in the United States of America by McNaughton and Gunn.

Library of Congress Cataloging-in-Publication Data:
Hull, Raymond H.
   Hearing and aging / Ray H. Hull.
      p. ; cm.
   Includes bibliographical references and index.
   ISBN-13: 978-1-59756-441-0 (alk. paper)
   ISBN-10: 1-59756-441-9 (alk. paper)
   I. Title.
   [DNLM: 1. Hearing Loss—etiology. 2. Hearing Loss—psychology. 3. Age
Factors. 4. Aged. 5. Hearing Aids. WV 270]
   LC classification not assigned
   617.8—dc23
                                             2011031834

Contents

Preface

This book is written for those who want a basic understanding of hearing loss that affects people as they age, and how they are served. Its purpose is to provide a basic look at the nature of hearing impairment as it manifests itself within the process of aging, the psychosocial-communicative impact of impaired hearing on the life of older adults, and a process for assisting older adults who are hearing impaired that can be used by both service providers including audiologists, and the family of the older adult.

The seven chapters of this book present information on: (1) the special nature of aging and the psychosocial impact of hearing impairment on older adults, (2) the aging auditory system, (3) the impact of hearing loss in older adulthood, (4) considerations on hearing aid use for older adults, (5) techniques for assisting older adults who possess impaired hearing, and (6) special considerations on the provision of services on behalf of confined older adults who reside in nursing homes and other types of health care facilities.

The appendixes identify resources that provide further information on hearing loss in aging, hearing aids, and considerations for serving older adults with impaired hearing. The reader will also find suggestions that will assist older adults with impaired hearing to function with greater efficiency in difficult listening environments.

The book is intended for use in the academic preparation of all who will serve older adults in a variety of settings, including those in audiology and speech-language pathology, nurses who are preparing to become geriatric nurse practice specialists, those who are preparing to become gerontologists, psychologists, family practice physicians, geriatric medicine specialists, and others who serve or who are preparing to serve older adults.

Because of the very practical nature of this book, it should prove to be a wonderful resource for family members and other significant persons in the lives of older adults who have impaired hearing. The information presented is often requested by many persons who know or serve older adults when the author speaks at conferences and conventions around the United States, Europe, and Canada.

Students will appreciate *Hearing and Aging* because it is clear and easy to read, and the content is practice-oriented rather than laden with philosophical discourse. Professionals who teach and/or practice in any field that serves older adults will enjoy it because it doesn't burden them with information that may not be topic-related, or cause them to feel guilty that their students were required to purchase a book that contains more information than was needed.

Hearing and Aging is designed to focus on the most important *practical* aspects for understanding the processes involved in assisting older adults with impaired hearing. It contains the material needed to understand the nature of hearing loss in older adulthood and the processes for serving those whose hearing is impaired. However, it avoids the technical detail of more cumbersome, theoretical texts.

This text provides students and professionals with concise and clearly readable information on the elements and processes for serving older adults with impaired hearing. Its beauty lies in its ease of reading which students, professionals, and lay persons will applaud. It is clear and readable in presentation. It is "holistic" in scope, and within its pages is a neatly presented eclectic approach to serving diverse populations of older adults. It is likely to receive accolades from students, professionals, and others who serve older adults with impaired hearing.

Ray H. Hull, PhD

Introduction

Older adults in most instances are no different from younger ones other than they have grown older. They have the same personality, perhaps a little stronger, but basically the same. They look the same except for some wrinkles and sagging skin, and perhaps are a little shorter due to the pull of gravity over the years. Their voice will be the same except for some change due to the aging vocal mechanism, so pitch may raise slightly, and they may speak a little louder due to a decline in hearing. Their walking gait may slow a little as they may not exercise as much as they used to and their joints might ache, and they may be wearing reading glasses because of a change in near vision. But, everyone is different, and some people age faster and more dramatically than others. When I was in my first year of graduate school, one of my classmates by the name of Bob, at age 23, was bald, white faced, somewhat prematurely wrinkled around the face, and had a voice that resembled that of an old man. In other words, he looked and acted "old." So, we all age differently. I like to think of myself as a younger/older person, but perhaps I am deluding myself.

One aspect of growing older that seems to be common is a change in hearing acuity and the ability to process what one hears with the speed and efficiency experienced in earlier years; therefore, the ability to hear and comprehend what the TV news broadcaster or spouse is saying may be steadily declining.

Hearing does decline with some regularity as the years pass. Our inner ears, which contain around 18,000 nerve receptors in our younger years, will probably not contain as many by age 70 years, so certain sounds of speech and music may not be heard as well. This is primarily because we live in a noisy world, and the tiny nerve receptors of our inner ears are not designed to withstand such punishment, so they die, particularly those that respond best to high-pitched sounds of speech and music. Furthermore, the centers of the brainstem and brain that are supposed to process what we hear with the speed necessary to permit us to understand what is being said may have difficulty keeping up with the many subtle sounds of speech and the language clues of human communication that generally are spoken so rapidly that few people can understand.

This book is designed to help readers understand the process of aging, its impact on human hearing, and the impact of impaired hearing in older people. Most importantly, it provides information on how to serve those whose hearing has declined over the years. I hope it helps you to understand the frustrations that approximately 70 million adults over age 50 years experience as a result of declining hearing, and some ideas on how to assist them in a world of people who do not speak as plainly as they should, and places that are not meant for communication.

CHAPTER 1

Hearing Loss in Older Adulthood

GABRIELLE SAUNDERS
DAWN KONRAD-MARTIN
RAY H. HULL

HEARING LOSS IN AGING:
THE PROBLEM AND IMPACT

Today's world is a busy and noisy place, filled with sounds, sights, and movement. Many older adults can find it difficult to process this incoming information and still concentrate on what people are saying. In terms of hearing, they often complain that the new generation "mumbles" and "talks too fast." Although this may sometimes be true, these difficulties can also be associated with the aging auditory system including the auditory areas of the brain. Changes in our ability to hear and understand as we

1

age are termed "presbycusis" which occurs as a result of exposure to noise, disease, certain medications, heredity, and the normal aging process.

Presbycusis results in decreased ability to hear high-pitched sounds such as [s], [sh], [f], and [th], and in a gradual slowing of our central nervous system's ability to process rapidly spoken speech with the speed and precision necessary to process what is heard. In our noisy busy world, this can lead to misunderstandings and frustration not only on the part of the older listener, but also on the part of friends and family of the person whose hearing and processing ability has changed. It is sometimes incorrectly assumed that their loved one is inattentive, or not listening properly.

The Impact

Presbycusis is a high-burden disorder that can have devastating effects on the older person, their family, and others with whom they interact. Presbycusis, like all forms of hearing impairment, reduces the ability to understand speech, particularly when in difficult listening situations such as when there is background noise or when the speaker talks fast. When untreated, this may isolate the sufferer from his or her family, friends, and society, resulting in depression, anxiety, and loneliness, as well as loss of confidence at work, decreased participation in social activities, and stress on intimate relationships (Kochkin & Rogin, 2000). Furthermore, individuals with hearing loss may be more likely to require the use of health care services (Ebert & Heckerling, 1995) and may exhibit more comorbid conditions than those without hearing impairment (Barnett & Franks, 1999; Gates, Cobb, D'Agostino, & Wolf, 1993). The spouse or significant other of a hearing-impaired person is also impacted by presbycusis; they often report irritation at having to be their partner's interpreter, report stress, anxiety, and feeling ill-at-ease when in public with their hearing-impaired spouse, and, like their partner, can become socially isolated (Hetu, Jones, & Getty, 1993).

Incidence of Hearing Loss in Older Adulthood

The incidence of hearing loss, especially among the elderly is considerable. Figure 1–1 shows data collected from almost 6,000 individuals aged 20 to 69 who took part in the National Health and Nutrition Examination Survey (Agrawal, Platz, & Niparko, 2008). The figure shows the percentage of the population for each cohort that has hearing loss, defined either as having a hearing loss greater than 25 dB HL for the lower and middle frequencies of 0.5, 1, and 2 kHz, or a hearing loss that is greater than 25 dB HL for the higher frequencies of 3, 4, and 6 kHz. It is seen that the prevalence of hearing loss rises with cross-sectional age, with greater prevalence rates found for the hearing loss definition that is based on higher frequencies. Similarly,

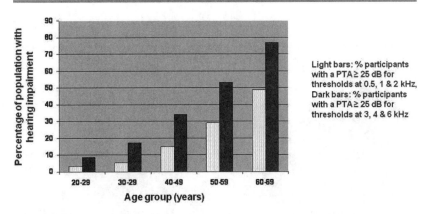

Light bars: % participants with a PTA≥ 25 dB for thresholds at 0.5, 1 & 2 kHz, Dark bars: % participants with a PTA≥ 25 dB for thresholds at 3, 4 & 6 kHz

FIGURE 1–1. Hearing loss incidence defined using a 0.5, 1, and 2-kHz pure-tone average (PTA) and a 3, 4, and 6-kHz PTA. Data from the 1994–2004 National Health and Nutrition Examination Survey. Data from Agrawal, Y., Platz, E., & Niparko, J. (2008). Prevalence of hearing loss and differences by demographic characteristics among U.S. adults. *Archives of Internal Medicine 168*(14), 1522–1530.

the Health, Aging, and Body Composition Study (Helzner et al., 2005) shows that almost 60% of individuals aged 73 to 84 years have hearing loss when it is defined as a pure-tone threshold average of 25 dB HL or greater for the frequencies of 0.5, 1, and 2 kHz, but when the definition of hearing loss includes thresholds at 3 and 4 kHz (frequencies critical for understanding speech) the incidence increases to almost 77%.

Longitudinal studies further document the decline of hearing with age. The rate of this decline is related to age and gender. In one large study, hearing threshold shifts averaged across age groups and gender for adults aged 60 and over was as follows: 0.7 dB per year for lower frequencies, increasing to 1.2 dB per year at 8 kHz and 1.23 dB per year at 12 kHz (Lee, Matthews, Dubmo, & Mills, 2005). As seen in Figure 1–2, the decline in men is greater in the higher frequencies than at low frequencies up to age 80 years. Lower frequency thresholds (0.5–2 kHz) changed at a lesser rate than the higher frequency thresholds for both sexes (Congdon et al., 2004). An important implication of these data is that hearing sensitivity at *all* frequencies, typically

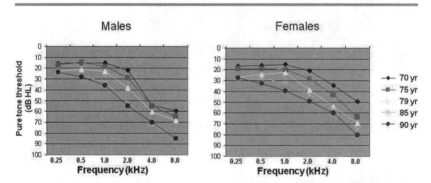

FIGURE 1–2. Progression of hearing loss with age. Data from the Gerontological and geriatric study (1971), Gotteborg, Sweden. Published by Jonsson, R, and Rosenthall, U. (1998). Hearing in Advanced Age. A study of Presbycusis in 85-, 88-, and 90-year-old people. *Audiology,* *37*(4), 207–218.

is abnormal in the later decades of life. These sensitivity changes almost certainly disrupt speech understanding and increase the need for hearing rehabilitation in the later decades of life.

The U.S. Census Bureau suggests there currently are almost 40 million people over age 65, with almost 6 million being over age 85 years. This translates to at least 31 million with hearing loss (Kochkin, 2005). It is projected that by 2050 there will be 88.5 million people over age 65 and that 19 million of these will be over age 85 years (U.S. Census Bureau, 2008), with the fastest growing population being those over age 100 years. Although there no readily available estimates of the economic cost of presbycusis, it is known that the average lifetime societal costs of severe to profound hearing loss in the United States are $297,000 per hearing-impaired individual (Mohr et al., 2000); thus, as the prevalence of presbycusis increases, so will its economic and social burden on society.

EFFECTS OF AGE ON HEARING ABILITIES

Presbycusis involves deficits at multiple sites within the auditory pathway. Contributions to presbycusis from specific peripheral and central auditory stages of processing are difficult to distinguish clinically, but it is important to do so as far as possible because the techniques appropriate for addressing cochlear dysfunction may be substantially different from those appropriate for addressing speech processing or cognitive deficits. Table 1–1 provides an overview of changes in hearing abilities that accompany aging. Also listed are the underlying types of processing, and the sites of lesion that these changes may implicate. The rationale for visualizing the auditory system in this way is to provide a systematic approach to clinical intervention.

Aging and Peripheral Auditory Function

Age-related changes in the function of the outer and middle ear are apparent from changes in the appearance of the outer ear and

TABLE 1–1. Hearing Ability Deficit, Associated Type of Processing, and Lesion Sites

Deficit in Hearing Ability	Type of Processing	Lesion Sites
Sounds are not audible	Auditory acuity and signal detection	External Ear, Middle Ear, and Inner Ear
Small operating range between sounds that can be just detected and those that are intolerably loud Frequency contrasts not detectable	Auditory acuity and signal detection	Inner Ear
Rapid changes in sound/complex acoustic features of signal not detectable	Neural processing and transmission	Auditory Nerve, Brain
Trouble storing and retrieving information Trouble coding, organizing, associating information	Working memory and attention Integration with existing linguistic and other mental constructs	Brain

the frequent observation of middle ear involvement at 4 kHz in older adults (Glorig & Davis, 1961). Effects of age are shown through a decrease in middle ear stiffness caused by changes in the elasticity of tissues (reviewed by Zafar, 1994; Feeney & Sanford, 2004). Outer and middle ear contributions to age-related sensitivity loss are considered relatively minor, but a common related problem is collapse of the ear canal during testing when using headphones for measuring hearing. This problem yields inaccurate thresholds and can be prevented by the use of insert earphones.

Age-related changes in the peripheral auditory system have been extensively studied, but it remains a challenge to separate effects of the normal aging process from exposure to external sources of damage in humans such as noise and disease. Changes to inner ear and auditory nerve function are thought to under-lie the decrease in hearing sensitivity that accompanies aging. In a series of famous studies Schuknecht and colleagues (e.g., Schucknecht, 1974; Schucknecht & Gacek, 1993), identified four types of inner ear presbycusis:

1. **Sensory presbycusis.** This profile was associated with atrophy and degeneration of the cochlear hair cells and supporting cells. Damage was greatest toward the basal, high-frequency coding end of the cochlea.

2. **Neural presbycusis.** Reduced size and number of spiral ganglion cells and auditory nerve fibers was found.

3. **Metabolic or strial presbycusis.** Degeneration of the cochlear lateral wall, and particularly of the stria vascularis was observed.

4. **Mechanical presbycusis.** Changes in physical properties of the cochlea were proposed to alter basilar membrane mechanics.

Neural and metabolic presbycusis are still considered common forms of the disorder. Sensory cell loss is almost certainly com-mon among older hearing-impaired adults, but primarily may reflect a lifetime of exposure to loud sounds, rather than aging per se. Most hearing losses are combinations of these pathologies and pure Schuknecht types are infrequently observed (Working Group on Speech Understanding and Aging of the Committee on Hearing Bioacoustics and Biomechanics, 1988). There also is evidence that metabolic presbycusis may be genetically deter-mined (Gates, Couropmitree, & Myers, 1999).

The Effects of Cochlear Degeneration

Damage to the cochlear outer hair cells influences both the audibility and understandability of speech. Specifically, the outer hair cell system provides frequency-specific amplification of low-level sound input, but also affects hearing by affording fine-frequency tuning and the ability to detect a wide range of sound intensities. Lack of frequency tuning reduces the ability to hear frequency contrasts within the speech signal, and so acts as a source of signal distortion.

The Effects of a Loss of Auditory Nerve Inputs to the Central Auditory Nervous System.

Perceptual consequences of a loss of auditory nerve inputs to the central auditory nervous system are hypothesized to include a reduction in the ability to process temporal cues (Zeng, Kong, Michalewski, & Starr, 2005). What this means is that the ability to follow rapid changes in the speech signal over time is degraded and the speech signal is more difficult to interpret.

Aging, Central Auditory Function, and Cognition

In an early study by Jerger (1972), the performance of young normal-hearing listeners, young hearing-impaired listeners, and older hearing-impaired listeners on four measures of speech understanding were measured. He found that the normal hearing listeners performed better than the two hearing-impaired groups, but that the older hearing-impaired listeners performed more poorly than the young listeners with the same degree of hearing impairment. In other words, the older listeners performed more poorly than their actual ability to hear would suggest. Since that time, other studies have shown that, as compared to younger listeners, the elderly have poorer performance on tests of speech processing (Gordon-Salant & Fitzgibbons, 2001), speech in noise (Plomp & Mimpen, 1979), and higher level language processing (Wingfield et al., 2006). The presence of auditory processing deficits combined with elevated thresholds, means the individual must use greater perceptual effort to process incoming sensory signals than normal, which likely explains why even mild-to-moderate hearing impairment affects memory (McCoy et al., 2005).

Brainstem and Brain

There are pronounced effects of age on the structure of the nerve cells of the brainstem and auditory cortex: the primary areas of the central nervous system responsible for speech understanding and comprehension. Postmortem studies of human brains show an age-related reduction in the number and size of neurons in the brainstem (Briner & Willot, 1989; Kirikae, Sato, & Shitara, 1964) and auditory cortex (Brody, 1955). Evidence for changes in brain neurochemistry that facilitate the timing mechanisms of the brain necessary for speech interpretation also has been found. Thus, these age-related changes in the central auditory system may contribute to speed and precision of processing and speech understanding deficits in the elderly.

Brain imaging studies suggest that, even when performance is matched between groups of older and younger adult subjects, older brains behave differently for a fairly broad range of tasks, including those that assess verbal and spatial working memory. Some studies show activity in regions of older brains that are not activated by the same task in younger brains (Grady & Craik, 2000; Reuter-Lorenz, 2002; Reuter-Lorenz, Jonides et al., 2000). That is, there appears to be a relative overactivation of prefrontal locations. This has led to the hypothesis that overactivity in older brains is related to the need for the brain to "work harder" to make up for reduced processing efficiency, or information that is masked or degraded by noise or by a degraded signal.

Studies have also shown greater activation in a similar region of the opposite hemisphere in the brains of older adults that is not present in the brains of younger adults. The many changes that accompany aging suggest that each older patient will be unique in terms of particular abilities, limitations, and rehabilitative needs.

NONAUDITORY BARRIERS TO COMMUNICATION AND AUDITORY REHABILITATION

Normal aging is accompanied by changes in all organs and systems of the body: eyes, hearing, taste, muscles, skin, brain, heart, and so forth. The relevance here is that some of these changes directly affect communication and the ability of older adults to respond to rehabilitation.

Aging, Vision Loss, and Communication

Vision loss is also common among the aging population. It is estimated that more than 3 million people aged 65 and older have some form of uncorrectable visual impairment (REF). Like hearing loss, the numbers increase dramatically with age (Figure 1–3).

Good vision is important for speech understanding and when absent it disrupts interpersonal communication. Visual cues from the lips and tongue of the speaker supplement speech understanding, especially when in a noisy environment. Walden, Busacco, and Montgomery (1993) illustrated this in a study of elderly participants. When these individuals listened to sentences presented in noise they scored about 43%; however, when these same individuals were able to watch the speaker's face at the same time, their scores increased to over 90%. Nonverbal visual cues such as gestures, facial expressions, posture, and

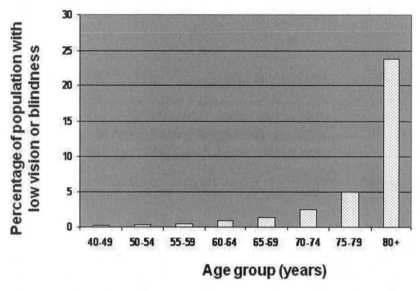

FIGURE 1–3. Percentage of population with uncorrectable visual impairment by age group.

eye contact also provide metalinguistic information: information about the speaker's mood and intent. When this information is unavailable the listener misses these subtle cues, which can lead to misunderstandings and miscommunication.

Aging, Cognition, and Communication

The auditory processing and cognitive processing deficits associated with aging that were described above have a variety of implications for interpersonal communication, particularly for the communication that takes place between clinical providers and their elderly patients, especially if the provider speaks quickly or when there are distractions present. More effort is required for older individuals to decode the incoming sensory input, leaving fewer resources for other aspects of speech understanding, such as thinking about the content of the speech or transferring the information into memory. As a consequence recall of information likely will be poorer and the patient may tire more quickly.

NONAUDITORY BARRIERS TO HEARING REHABILITATION

Typically, auditory rehabilitation consists of at least three visits to the audiologist, although some audiologists provide additional rehabilitation in the form of group auditory rehabilitation counseling sessions, at which additional communication strategies and problems are discussed. At the first visit, the patient's hearing is evaluated, their needs are discussed, a rehabilitation plan is devised, and assistive technology (usually hearing aids) ordered. At the second visit, the hearing aids may be fitted, information about their use and upkeep is provided, and strategies for communication are discussed. At the third visit, the audiologist assesses whether the patient is having success with the hearing aids, and the hearing output needs to be fine-tuned to optimize sound quality.

In just three visits short visits then, a considerable amount of information is exchanged. It therefore is critical that the audiologist optimizes communication with the patient, and that the audiologist and patient work closely together to select the auditory rehabilitation most likely to lead to success in terms of effectiveness and patient satisfaction. How can this be best achieved and what are the key points to consider? Below we discuss some of these.

Communication Needs

The lifestyles and needs of the elderly population are varied, ranging from those individuals who maintain a job, an active social life, and are involved with their community, to those with poor health whose communication needs are limited to a caregiver, the telephone, and the television. The assistive technology provided should reflect the patient's communication needs. This might mean selecting a high-end hearing aid and personal FM system for the active individual, or a personal amplifier for the television and an in-line telephone amplifier for the individual whose life is limited to their home. There are questionnaires, such as the Client Oriented Scale of Improvement (Dillon, James, & Ginis, 1997) and the Glasgow Hearing Aid Benefit Profile (Gatehouse, 1999) that ask patients to specify the listening situations of most importance to them. These questionnaires take only a few minutes to complete, and provide an easy way for the audiologist to ensure they are addressing at least some of the patient's needs.

Hearing Aids

Hearing aids cannot restore hearing to normal. At their most basic they amplify sounds, and thus make quiet sounds more audible. At their most sophisticated they can address loudness growth issues and directionality. However, currently no hearing aid can truly compensate for cochlear damage or changes in auditory processing ability that diminish the clarity of speech, although by increasing audibility more brain-processing resources are made available for decoding and recall. Indeed, studies show hearing aids to be a successful form of intervention. For example, the National Counsel on the Aging (Kochkin & Rogin, 2000) study of over 2,000 hearing-impaired individuals found that hearing instruments resulted in improved interpersonal relationships, reduced anger and frustration, reduced depression, depressive symptoms, and anxiety, enhanced emotional stability, increased earning power, decreased social phobias and self-criticism, enhanced group social activity, and improved cognitive function.

Hearing aids come in different shapes and sizes. The needs and lifestyle of the user, the user's ability to manipulate a hearing aid, and visual ability should impact the style and features of the hearing aid selected. For example, an individual with good fine-motor skills, good visual acuity, and an active lifestyle might be best suited to a hearing aid with sophisticated signal processing capabilities. On the other hand, someone with a more limited lifestyle who also has poor annual dexterity due to a degenerative disease like Parkinson disease would likely not use sophisticated processing features and would be unable to insert any hearing aid unless it is relatively large. Similarly, a visually impaired individual may also encounter difficulties changing the batteries and seeing tiny hearing aid switches. It is the audiologist's responsibility to help patients select hearing aids with features they need, and with controls they can handle and see.

Patient-Provider Communication

Good communication between the patient and the audiologist is key to a successful outcome. As outlined above, hearing loss, vision loss, and the effects of cognitive aging all can compromise success. There are a number of relatively simple ways to improve communication with the older patient. They can be divided into those associated with optimizing the physical environment and those associated with behavioral changes during communication, as listed below.

1. **Environmental Accommodations:**

   ▉ Face the patient to increase likelihood of him or her being able to see your face and lips

   ▉ Keep the office space bright. Use incandescent lighting

   ▉ Do not sit in front of a window as backlighting makes your face more difficult to see.

   ▉ Make sure there are no moving distractions nearby, such as a window that looks out onto a busy reception area, or a TV screen

   ▉ Have a magnifying glass available for showing patients small objects or written materials.

2. Behavioral Accommodations:

■ Get the patient's attention *and* establish eye-contact before beginning any discussion

■ Speak slowly and clearly but do not exaggerate sounds and do not shout. Shouting distorts the auditory signal and exaggeration distorts transitions between phonemes, making them more difficult to understand

■ Repeat and emphasize key points, but avoid providing unnecessary information

■ Inform the patient when the topic of discussion is going to change. For example, "Now that you have told me about your hearing loss, we are going to move on to talking about some possible ways to help you"

■ Suggest to patients that they have a family member or friend accompany them to their visit. The more people listening, the more likely it is that someone will recall the information provided

■ Provide written materials summarizing the key points discussed during the visit to reinforce the information. The patient can take these home to read in a nonstressful environment. Some guidance based on a publication from the Centers for Disease Control and Prevention & Agency for Toxic Substances and Disease Registry (1999) for developing readable materials is provided in Table 1–2.

SUMMARY

When one considers the prevalence of hearing impairment among the older population, the physical changes that accompany aging, and the impacts that communication deficits have on daily function and quality of life, it should become clear that

TABLE 1–2. Developing Readable Materials for Use in the Treatment of Older Adults

Content	Formatting	Printing
Include only critical information	Use 14-point font or larger	Print on nonglossy paper
Avoid long lists	Put key information at the start and end of the brochure	Use contrasting colors, e.g., black on white
Make concrete statements	Use informative headings to chunk the information	Keep pictures simple. Annotate them with bold arrows to explain the point of each.
Use short sentences	Use bullets not ongoing text	Use a simple font. Avoid big curlicues, etc.
Use positive statements, e.g., "Keep your hearing aid dry," as opposed to "Do not get your hearing aid wet"	Do not justify the right margin	Leave lots of white space between text and pictures
State up front the purpose of the material, e.g., "This booklet tells you how to look after your hearing aids"	Use columns of about 40–50 characters.	
Use vocabulary and sentence structure of Grade 8 and below		

recognition and management of hearing impairment is critical. The clinician should consider individual differences among older patients when selecting interventions. Peripheral impairments in part can be addressed with hearing aids, to the extent that hearing aids are able to make most speech sounds audible. Central and cognitive processing impairments can be addressed through the use of an FM device combined with some form of auditory training, whereas some behavioral and comorbid conditions can be addressed though counseling and wise choices on the part of the clinician. However, we still do not have a complete understanding of the underlying physiological and psychological changes associated with aging, nor do we have solutions to many of the rehabilitative needs of this growing population. This highlights the need for ungoing research in this field.

CHAPTER 2

The Impact of Impaired Hearing on Older Adults

INTRODUCTION

It is clear that the effects of aging on individuals are as unique as their response to the process. But, when the effects of aging begin to impact negatively on sensory processes that previously permitted efficient personal and social functioning, then it may become even more difficult to cope with advancing age. The sensory deficit discussed earlier in this book is presbycusis, or hearing impairment as a result of the process of aging.

THE IMPACT

Whatever the cause of the disorder called presbycusis, or how it is manifested, the effects on the some 24 million older adults who possess it, in many respects, are the same. The disappointment of not having been able to understand what their children and grandchildren were saying at the last family reunion can be frustrating, to say the least. It becomes easier to withdraw from situations where communication with others may take place rather than face embarrassment from frequent misunderstandings of statements and inappropriate responses. To respond to the question, "How did you sleep last night?" with "At home, of course!" is embarrassing, particularly when other misinterpretations may have occurred within the same conversation and continue with increasing regularity. An older adult who otherwise may be an alert, intelligent individual will understandably be concerned about such misunderstandings. Many older adults who experience such difficulties feel that perhaps they are "losing their mind," particularly when they may not know the cause for the speech understanding problems. Perhaps their greatest concern is that their family may feel that they are losing the ability to function independently and that the personal aspects of life for which they are responsible will be taken away.

Communication is such an integral part of financial dealings, for example, that older adults may also question their own ability to maintain a responsible position in the family, although in the end they may not wish to withdraw from those responsibilities. The self-questioning that may occur can be further aggravated by well-meaning comments by others. A comment by a concerned son or daughter such as, "Dad, why don't you think about selling the house and moving into an apartment? You know this house is too much for you to care for," can be disquieting. Even though an older family member may be adequately caring for the house, cooking nutritious meals, and looking forward to each spring so that he or she can work in the garden, a seed of doubt about one's ability to maintain a house and other life requirements adequately because of age has been planted. A statement by his or her physician such as, "Of course you're having aches and pains, you're no spring chicken any more," can bring about doubts of survival.

Compounding these self-doubts may be a growing inability to understand what others are saying because of presbycusis. It becomes easier, for lack of other alternatives, to withdraw from communicative situations in which embarrassment or fear of embarrassment may occur. If forced into such a difficult situation, the easiest avenue is to become noncommunicative rather than to attempt responses to questions and fail, thus instilling doubts in younger family members' minds about one's ability to maintain independent living. If forced into responding to questions that are not fully understood because an important word is missed or misunderstood, frustration by both the older adult and the family can result.

How Do Older Adults React to Their Hearing Impairment?

Feelings of embarrassment, frustration, anger, and ultimate withdrawal from situations that require communication are very real among older adults who possess impaired hearing and those who interact with them. When so much else is taken away from many older adults including leadership in their family, a steady income, a spouse or friend who may have recently passed away, convenient transportation, and a regular social life, a gradual decrease in one's ability to hear and understand what others are saying can be debilitating. As one elderly adult told this author, "I would like to participate socially, but I feel isolated when I cannot hear."

Many older adults feel so frustrated by their inability to understand what the minister is saying at church, what their friends are saying at the senior center, or what the speaker at an anticipated meeting is saying, that they cease attending. They may be described by their family or others with whom they associate as noncommunicating, uncooperative, withdrawn, and, most unkind of all, "confused or senile." A less than expected benefit from the use of hearing aids may further result in fear by the older adult or his or her family that, perhaps, the disorder is mental rather than auditory.

It has been observed by this author that, in some instances, a portion of the depression experienced by older persons who have impaired hearing is brought about by feelings that break-downs in communication being experienced "are all my fault because it is my hearing impairment." It may not occur to them that the disorder of hearing may be magnified by family members who do not speak plainly, or by being placed in communicative environments that are so noisy and otherwise distracting that persons with normal auditory function are also having difficulty hearing and understanding the speech of others. For example, those may include attempting to listen to a speaker in an auditorium with poor acoustics when the only seat left upon arrival was toward the rear of the room under the balcony; watching a 20-year-old television set with a distorted signal; or attempting to understand what his or her shy 3-year-old grand-daughter is saying.

Some older adults who have hearing impairment become so defeated in their attempts at communication that it does not occur to them that they might be better able to understand what others are saying if those with whom they are communicating would either improve their manner of speaking, or improve the communicative environment. However, many older adults have resigned themselves to "not be a bother" rather than assert themselves by criticizing their family's manner of speaking or the environments in which they are asked to communicate. Rather, older adults may simply visit their families less frequently, even though they desire to be with their daughter or son and grand-children. Sadly, however, they may withdraw into isolation at home rather than attempt to maintain social or family contacts where they previously have felt frustration and embarrassment.

How Do Others React to Older Adults Who Possess Hearing Impairment?

One 82-year-old adult quite eloquently stated to this author, "For every poor ear, there's at least one poor speaker and one noisy place where it is difficult to understand what I am supposed to be hearing!" He was probably quite accurate in his appraisal, or perhaps even understated it.

As stated earlier, many older adults have placed themselves in a position of "not being a bother," perhaps not realizing that at least a portion of their difficulties in communication with others may be the result of attempting to talk to persons who do not speak clearly or being asked to communicate in environments that may cause even a person with normal hearing to have difficulty. However, even though an older person's adult child may lack good speech skills, the blame for miscommunication or misunderstanding by the elderly parent with hearing impairment may be placed on them, and not the speaker, without attempting to analyze ways to enhance interpersonal communication.

Generally, the initial visible frustration with an older adult's inability to understand what is being said is noticed by a listener. A lesser reaction may have resulted in a simple request for repetition or rephrasing of the statement for clarification. When an elderly listener with hearing impairment fails to understand a statement after several repetitions of a difficult word, it is usually he or she who first notices the apparent frustration on the face of the speaker, rather than the speaker her or himself. Increased self-imposed pressure to succeed in understanding a problem word within a speaker's sentence tends to increase anxiety and heighten the probability of failure to understand it. One of two reactions generally follows: (1) The most frequent on the part of an elderly listener is to become frustrated, apologize, and withdraw. (2) The second probable response is a feeling of anger coupled with frustration and embarrassment and either a covert or overt expression of, "Why don't you speak more clearly!"

Where Does the Fault Lie?

Who initiated this trying situation? In all probability it was the *speaker* rather than the listener. The speaker's initial unspoken display of frustration at the older listener's inability to understand the statement or question may have caused heightened anxiety on the listener's part. Anxiety, in that situation, breeds failure, failure breeds frustration, frustration breeds further failure, and on and on, until some resolution to cease the conversation, leave the situation, or continue to display anger and frustration is reached.

Did the initial attempt at the conversation prompt this less than tolerable situation? Probably not. The person with impaired hearing who has been frustrated in attempting to hold conversations on previous occasions usually develops a fairly immediate awareness of signs of anxiety, frustration, or concern that are reflected in a speaker when a non-understood word or phrase leads to a delay or void in the conversation. After failure in various communicative environments on other occasions with other speakers, and perhaps occurring with greater regularity, the older adult begins to anticipate a speaker's response, perhaps prematurely in some instances. In any event, a speaker at some time has planted the seed of suspicion that he or she was frustrated, concerned, and perhaps even angry at the older listener's failure to understand or interpret what he or she was saying.

The second party's negative response to the older person's obvious difficulty in understanding what he or she is saying may be the result of an unanticipated interruption in the flow of a conversation. Otherwise, the reasons may be a lack of desire to really communicate with the older person, a lack of tolerance for a disorder that is not readily visible and therefore disconcerting to the unimpaired person, or a lack of knowledge regarding ways in which the situation could be made more comfortable for both the listener who has hearing impairment and the speaker.

An unimpaired person typically will assist a person who has difficulty walking to safely cross a busy street or guide a person who is visually impaired through a maze of chairs. In that situation, however, the impairment and the manner in which assistance can be offered are both obvious to a person who, in fact, may know little about the handicapping effects of blindness. But verbal communication, which generally is experienced as a rather smooth ongoing set of events, when interrupted by a invisible disorder such as hearing impairment, may be disconcerting to the unimpaired person. This can be true particularly when a hearing aid is not worn or otherwise displayed.

Communication for a brief instant no longer exists. At that point the person with unimpaired hearing may not know how to resolve the situation. The misunderstood word or phrase is repeated, but perhaps to no avail. The person who has impaired hearing may still misinterpret the verbal message. A natural response is to repeat the word or phrase once again in a louder voice, perhaps with emphasis and facial expression that reveals at least some frustration, as the speaker may not yet have determined why the listener is having difficulty understanding what he or she is saying. The evident frustration, in turn, may concern the listener who has impaired hearing, and communication is at a standstill.

If Hearing Loss Was More Noticeable

If the impaired auditory system of a person with impaired hearing was as noticeable as the impaired limbs of a person with a physical injury, perhaps the perplexing frustrations that occur could be reduced. Presbycusis is such a complex auditory disorder, however, that simply raising the intensity of one's voice may do little to ease the difficulty. In fact, in some instances, the misinterpretations can actually increase as a result of heightened anxiety. In other words, the frustrations experienced by both persons who possess unimpaired hearing and those with impaired hearing do exist, and can negatively influence communication when solutions on how to reduce the communication breakdowns are not known.

Hearing-Impaired Older Adults Versus Others Who Are Hearing-Impaired

Why do family members, friends, or spouses of elderly adults with presbycusis appear to be more frustrated than persons who, for example, must communicate with children who have impaired hearing? Adults and children, perhaps, tend to be more compassionate toward children and young adults who have difficulty communicating as the result of hearing impairment. That is not to say that there are not instances in which attempts at getting a message across to a child who has impaired hearing fail in frustration for both the child and the speaker. Accommodations by unimpaired children and adults, however, appear to be made willingly in most instances because they know a child is likely to have difficulty understanding their verbal message, either because of the hearing impairment per se or as the result of language delay. On the other hand, the unimpaired person who is frustrated at attempts to communicate with an elderly adult who has impaired hearing may rationalize the reason as because the person is simply "old."

Are the frustrations and resulting tension expressed because a listener is an older person? Perhaps in a few instances this may be true, but probably not as a general rule. Frustrations of persons who may have known an elderly person for some time before the onset of the auditory difficulties may be because this person "was always quite alert." For reasons unknown to them, however, frustrating and failed attempts at "communicating with Dad" are causing friction within their family. "Dad's mind seems to be failing. I told him yesterday to get the safety inspection sticker for his car renewed and he asked, 'Who was safe?' Maybe we should get him a hearing aid." When a hearing aid is purchased for this elder by a well-meaning son or daughter, but he refuses to wear it because, as he says, "It doesn't help," he then may be described by his family as stubborn. Or they may feel that, "He refuses to do anything to improve himself," when in reality perhaps the hearing aid did not provide significant improvement because it was not selected and fit in accordance with the configuration of his hearing and his auditory needs.

So, how do others who associate with the elderly person with presbycusis react to him or her? As one family member said to this writer:

> We are concerned about Dad. We used to have a good time talking about things we are all interested in, and about what he wanted to do after he retired. Now that he can't seem to hear us or understand what we say, we all get angry. He can't understand what we are saying no matter how loud we talk,

and all he does is get mad because no matter how many times we repeat what we say, he still can't get it. We bought him a hearing aid, but he won't wear it. He says it doesn't help. For $2500, it should do something for him, but we all feel that he just can't get used to something new. Besides, he's just stubborn, we think. Our whole lives have changed since this hearing problem has gotten worse. We don't communicate anymore. We don't even like to have him over, and no one goes to visit him. He just sits. We are embarrassed to take him out to restaurants because he can't understand the waiters and then becomes angry when we try to interpret what they are saying. And, he talks so loud! So we just let him sit at his house. We told him to sell the house and move into an apartment complex where other older persons live. He says that if we try to sell his house he'll lock the doors and windows and never come out until the hearse takes him away. His hearing problem has changed all of our lives for the worse. We really are at our wits' end!

Such statements by concerned and frustrated children, friends, and spouses of older persons who have hearing impairment are heard numerous times in the audiologist's professional life. But the vast majority of these older adults can be helped if those who serve them take the time to listen to their responses to their auditory disorder and their state in life, and to have the hearing disorder carefully evaluated. From this information, viable service programs can be developed, not only for older persons who have hearing impairment, but also for those who most closely associate with them.

REACTIONS BY OLDER ADULTS TO THEIR HEARING IMPAIRMENT: A DIALOGUE

How do older adults with impaired hearing react to the disorder and the difficulties they have in attempting to communicate with others? The following statements from patients reflect their feelings about their hearing loss. They are taken from initial pretreatment interviews with 10 older adults who have impaired hearing and were video-recorded by this author. This type of personalized information provides important insights into the feelings and desires of older adults that are not only important in the counseling process, but also in the development of treatment programs on their behalf.

Case Studies: The Interviewees

All of the interviewees are of an average socioeconomic level and are bright, articulate older adults. All, however, possess a frustrating impairment of hearing.

Occupational History

Two women were teachers, one at the elementary and the other at high school level. One man managed a grain elevator in a rural community. He had no formal education past the sixth grade. One man was a retired agricultural agent for Weld County, CO. One man was a farmer, with no formal education past the eighth grade. Four women still consider themselves to be housewives and not retired. One man was a retired missionary. Four of these individuals presently reside in health care facilities, and the remainder are living in the community in their own homes.

State of Health and Mobility

The six adults interviewed who reside in the community all described themselves as being well. They described themselves as mobile, although only one of the women drove a car. All of the men who do not reside in a health care facility drive their own car. The women who were not driving a car said that transportation occasionally was a problem, but that city bus service was generally adequate, or friends or relatives would take them where they wanted to go. All patients interviewed, except one man who was troubled with gout, stated that they sometimes walked where they needed to go, mostly for exercise.

No patients interviewed who resided in health care facilities drove a car. Transportation was stated generally as being adequate through local bus service or by the health care facility's "ambulobus" service. The adults who reside in health care facilities generally described the reason for placement there as health reasons, except for one who felt that she was simply deposited there. Health and physical problems among those confined persons included heart problems, kidney dysfunction, Parkinson disease, visual impairments, and hearing loss. Walking was described by all as somewhat difficult. Two patients were confined to wheelchairs: one because of Parkinson disease and one because of arthritis.

Age

Ages of the patients included here ranged from 74 to 95 years. The mean age was 81 years.

Reason for Referral

All persons interviewed for this discussion had been referred for aural rehabilitation services or had sought out the service. All had consented to participate in aural rehabilitation treatment on an individual or group basis after an initial hearing evaluation and counseling.

The Dialogue

The following are the interviewees' descriptions of themselves and the impact of their hearing impairment on them. Again, the dialogue is taken from video-recorded responses by each interviewee to the question, "How do you feel about yourself at this time and your ability to communicate with others?"

Video-recorded interviews are routinely held with each patient seen by this author prior to aural rehabilitation services and again at the program's conclusion. The purpose for all pre- and post-video-recorded interviews is to allow patients to confront themselves and their feelings about their ability to function in their communicating worlds. Changes in their opinions of themselves and their ability to function communicatively are thus more easily shown. Through this venue, patients are further allowed the opportunity to note changes in themselves and their opinions of their ability to communicate with others by watching and listening to their own statements.

The following are brief but descriptive excerpts of statements by patients.

Case 1

Age: 76

Sex: Female

Residence: Community (In own house)

Marital status: Never married

Prior occupation: Elementary educator

Health: Good

Mobility: Good

Dialogue

"I try to say, 'What did you say?' but sometimes they begin to appear angry. I become frustrated—so frustrated that I then become angry at myself, because I have become angry at those with whom I am talking. Do other people have problems where they cannot understand what people are saying? Am I the only one?"

"I didn't realize why I had begun to dislike going to meetings until I realized I was not hearing and understanding what they were saying. I had been blaming my friends—and they had been secretly blaming me. I hope I can retain their friendship after I explain to them that the problems weren't all their fault."

Discussion

This woman's comments indicate concern over the difficulties she is experiencing in her attempts at interacting with others. However, she is not resigned to continued failure. She is still striving to retain friendships with others. Furthermore, she is still enrolled in aural rehabilitation treatment and making satisfactory progress in learning to make positive change in her difficult communication environments.

Case 2

Age: 77 years

Sex: Female

Residence: Health care facility

Marital status: Widow

Prior occupation: Housewife

Health: Arthritis, renal disease

Mobility: Confined to wheelchair. Mobility severely limited.

Dialogue

"I feel handicapped. Anymore, I don't know what the demands are, or what capabilities I have. I try so hard to hear that I become very tired. I may pass away any day. Is there hope for me? I want to talk to my children more than anything else, but they are so busy and can't come to see me very often. I want to hear what the minister here is saying at the chapel. Church means a great deal to me now."

"I feel so alone when I can't participate in things I want to do. I can't weed out what I want to hear from the noises around me. The most important thing is communication. I desperately want it. My grandchildren—I pray that I can someday spend a pleasant afternoon with them."

Discussion

This woman feels despondent. She is, however, an alert person and desires that her situation will improve. She is enrolled in an aural rehabilitation treatment program, but her state of depression has not improved significantly. She says that if her family would visit her, it would help. Most importantly, she desires to have someone with whom to communicate on a daily basis.

Case 3

Age: 78 years

Sex: Male

Residence: Community (in own house)

Marital status: Widower

Prior occupation: Grain elevator manager

Health: Generally good. Has cardiovascular problems. Some dizziness noted on occasion.

Mobility: Good. Drives own car and is physically mobile. He is mentally alert and always seems to have a joke for the occasion. But, in most respects, he is a man of few words.

Dialogue

"It's embarrassing. When people find out that you have trouble hearing, they don't seem to want to talk to you anymore. If you ask them to speak up, sometimes they look angry."

"I feel that time is lost when I go to a meeting I have looked forward to going to and I can't understand a word they are saying. Most people do not seem to have good speech habits. On the other hand, my poor hearing doesn't help a bit either."

"My main goal in coming here is to learn to hear a woman's voice better, maybe a woman's companionship won't be so hard to come by. As they say, a woman's voice may not be as pretty as the song of a bird, but it's awful darn close!"

Discussion

This man possesses a significant speech recognition deficit, and strongly desires that aural rehabilitative services be of help to him. He feels that he has much to live for and is willing to work to improve his auditory/communication problems. Assertiveness training and manipulation of his communicative environments has supported these efforts.

Case 4

Age: 95 years

Sex: Female

Residence: Health care facility

Marital status: Widow

Prior occupation: Housewife

Health: Parkinson disease

Mobility: Severely limited. Is confined to a wheelchair.

Dialogue

"I would like to be free, to drive, to go visit children and friends. I would like to get away from confinement. I would like to be able to hear again—to be able to be a part of the conversations that take place in this home. It would be pleasant to hear the minister again or to talk to my children. They live far away, though, and can't come to visit."

"My main concern is death right now. I know that the infirmity I have will end in death. I don't know if I'm ready. If I could hear the minister here at this facility, maybe I would know."

Discussion

These comments are typical of many elderly persons who are confined to a health care facility. They feel many needs, but so few can easily be fulfilled. This woman is alert, however, and can respond to aural rehabilitation services including the use of hearing aids or other assistive listening devices so that she can more efficiently hear what the staff is saying, and importantly, the chaplain of the health care facility. And, if accommodations can be made in the chapel so that she can participate in those services, then one of her other desires would be fulfilled. Furthermore, if learning to manipulate her more difficult communicative environments can be achieved so that she can function better within the confines of the health care facility, then her remaining years will be less isolating.

Case 5

Age: 78 years

Sex: Male

Residence: Health care facility (Posthospitalization)

Marital status: Married

Prior occupation: County extension agent

Health: Intestinal blockage. Arthritis. Otherwise in generally good health.

Mobility: Generally good. Drives own car on occasion. Walks to many places.

Dialogue

"I feel lost sometimes. If I look at people right straight in the eye, then sometimes I get what they say. I get angry sometimes, but I've finally figured out that for every poor ear, there's at least one poor speaker!"

"It's rough to have poor ears. I have trouble hearing women's voices. I wish I could hear them, since I'm around women more now than ever before. Maybe it's me, maybe I don't have good attention.

"I wish I could hear my preacher. I go to church each Sunday, but I don't get much out of it."

"I wish I could understand what people are saying in a crowd, like when our children and our grandchildren come back home to visit. If I'm talking to only one person, sometimes I do okay."

Discussion

This man expresses a great many "wishes," but so far has not extended himself a great deal in aural rehabilitation services. In other words, he desires to improve, but seems to feel that either he does not possess the capability to regain greater communication function, or simply does not want to put forth the effort. He appears to have great communicative needs, but does not yet seem to be convinced that he can improve. Counseling is important here, accompanied by the fitting of hearing instruments or other assistive listening devices so that he can communicate more efficiently with others, watch television, and hear the sermons at church.

Case 6

Age: 74

Sex: Male

Residence: Community (in own house)

Marital status: Widower

Prior occupation: Farmer

Health: Excellent, except for gout, which restricts his mobility.

Mobility: Not as mobile as desired, because of the gout. Drives his own car and is an avid fisherman.

Dialogue

"In a crowd—I have my worst trouble. Riding in a car drives me crazy! One thing that I have found is that people don't talk with their mouth open. My ears hum, and that hurts too in terms of my ability to understand what people are saying. Some people talk with their hands in front of their mouth; that is very disturbing. I don't think that my children understand that my problem is my hearing—not my mind. It just seems like the voices don't come through. I went to the doctor and he says my hearing is ruined. My hearing is my only handicap. My minister has an English brogue and I can't understand a word of what he is saying! And, groups sound kind of like a beehive. I feel embarrassed. Someone speaks to you and you give them the wrong answer. I like to go to social gatherings, but I still get embarrassed. However, I certainly am not going to give up!"

Discussion

This man represents the almost ideal older patient for aural rehabilitation services. He is alert and active and desires to maintain himself as an active social person. He has also found a female companion who, like him, is an avid fisherman. What an ideal motivational factor for success in aural rehabilitation!

Case 7

Age: 81 years

Sex: Male

Residence: Community (in own house with spouse)

Marital status: Married

Prior occupation: Missionary. Still functions as part-time minister for a local church. He receives many requests to serve on community and church committees.

Health: Excellent

Mobility: Excellent. Walks a great deal and drives own car.

Dialogue

"My greatest concern is my inability to participate in council meetings at church. In some cases, I am in charge of the meeting, but if I cannot understand what the members are saying, then my participation is made almost impossible. It distresses me tremendously that in some instances I cannot perform my duties. Maybe it's me? Maybe my concentration wanders. Maybe my mind is not working as well now, although I feel that it is. I have 20 to 30 members in the Sunday school class that I teach. I find that I have terrible problems determining what their questions are. If I do not know what their questions are, how can I respond to their needs?"

Discussion

These statements are made by an obviously frustrated man. "How can I respond to their needs?" This man has a great deal to offer his community and church, but is beginning to feel defeated. The audiologist must consider this type of older patient as a high priority and intervene as a strategist to assist the person in learning what can be done to function more efficiently in his prioritized communicative environments. This includes counseling, learning to manipulate his communicative environments to his advantage, hearing aids, and others.

Case 8

Age: 83 years

Sex: Female

Residence: Community (In own house with spouse)

Marital status: Married

Prior occupation: Nonretired housewife

Health: Excellent

Mobility: Excellent, but has never learned to drive a car. Depends on husband or bus for transportation. Walks a great deal.

Dialogue

"My hearing loss has been a handicap to me. I ask people to speak up, and they sigh and sometimes I feel terribly embarrassed. Sometimes they shout at me, which hurts in more ways than one."

"I do wish people would speak more distinctly. Even with my family, they sometimes forget to speak up 'for Mom.'"

"On the telephone I tell people that I'm wearing a hearing aid whether I am or not. They usually speak up more after that."

"My husband says I am a different person in this later age. I used to be full of fun, but now I don't even want to go to church. I don't like to go because I don't understand what others including the minister are saying."

"It isn't all peaches and cream to be this way. It hurts more than anything when people laugh at you when you give the wrong answer to something they say. I just go home and cry."

"People mumble when they talk."

"I just sometimes want to get out of people's way. I don't want to be a bother to anyone — be a nuisance. I've lost my self-confidence and I don't know if I'll ever get it back."

Discussion

This otherwise vital woman was on the verge of giving up. Further, her husband was talking about placing her in a nursing home. After 15 weeks of individual aural rehabilitation treatment, with a great deal of motivational counseling, she learned to manipulate the majority of the communicative environments that were most difficult for her. Furthermore, after being fit with appropriate hearing aids, she has rejoined a women's social group from which she had previously resigned membership. The gradual progression from a depressed woman to one with renewed hope has been rewarding to observe.

Case 9

Age: 76 years

Sex: Female

Residence: Community (In own house)

Marital status: Single

Prior occupation: Elementary educator

Health: Excellent

Mobility: Excellent

Dialogue

"I was feeling concerned in as much as when people would ask me a question, I would know they were speaking, but I couldn't make sense out of it. I was afraid that my mind was going. I felt closed in, not comfortable—like I could hear, but little of it made sense—like I was losing my mind!"

"I think sometimes that people want me to go away. When I found out that my problem was with my hearing and not my mind, the relief was wonderful. Now I feel that I have something I can try to handle, where before I didn't think I had a chance."

"If people will bear with me, I'll be able to talk with them. I'm going to stay in there just as long as I can."

Discussion

This woman benefited greatly from initial counseling sessions regarding her auditory problem and learning some reasons for the difficulties she was encountering. After she found that the communicative problems she was experiencing were, "not the result of her mind," but rather her hearing, she was a ready candidate for a formal aural rehabilitation treatment program including the evaluation for and fitting of hearing aids, environmental design modifications, and others that were important to her treatment plan.

Case 10

Age: 79 years

Sex: Female

Residence: Health care facility. Stated that she thought her daughter was looking for an apartment for her, but found herself in the health care facility instead.

Marital status: Widow

Prior occupation: Housewife (nonretired)

Health: Generally excellent except for broken hip 2 years ago

Mobility: Somewhat restricted because of fear of falling. Otherwise excellent. She takes the bus to places she desires to go.

Dialogue

"I used to blame others for my inability to hear and understand what was being said, but someone the other day told me it was my fault, me and my inability to hear."

"A speaker at a meeting the other evening spoke for 45 minutes and I did not understand a word she was saying! The disturbing thing was that she refused to use the microphone!"

"I was in a car with two friends the other day; I rode in the back seat. They were talking in the front seat. They were talking about a person I had not seen for quite a while. They said something about a ball game, and something about Omaha, and something about someone becoming very ill. I finally felt that I had to say something, so I asked, 'She is well, isn't she?' Well, what they had said was that my friend had died! She became very ill during a ball game in Omaha and died while being taken by ambulance to the hospital. It was terribly embarrassing, but they don't become angry with me. It is frustrating to try to do well, but fail. I try not to be irritable. I think I can overcome it."

Discussion

This is an example of an alert, intelligent woman who, because of factors beyond her control, fell resulting in a broken hip and leg, and found herself unable to provide for her personal-physical needs. She was thus placed in a health care facility, one hopes for a relatively short time. She has only accepted such placement because of the evident short stay. She is responding well to aural rehabilitation treatment services, particularly in learning to cope within her most difficult environments and those with whom she must communicate. She has analyzed the reasons for many of her communicative difficulties, and is aware of her limitations.

SUMMARY

Auditory deficits as the result of presbycusis are as real as the people who possess the disorder. The disorder, however, affects each person in unique ways. One common denominator is evident, namely, that the resulting communication problems can be frustrating and, in many instances, debilitating. The most common strain among the confessions of these older persons involves the isolation and loneliness that they experience.

CHAPTER 3

Facilitating Psychological Adjustment to Impaired Hearing

R. STEVEN ACKLEY
RAY H. HULL[1]

INTRODUCTION

As stated by Kaplan (2001), the sense of hearing is integrally related to communication and interaction with other people, as people generally relate to others through verbal communication. For the majority of adults who are deaf or hard of hearing,

---

[1]The information in this chapter is an adaptation from a chapter in Hull (2010) *Introduction to Aural Rehabilitation*.

impairment of the sense of hearing means that the ability to interact communicatively with others may also be impaired. The frustrations that arise from misinterpreted verbal messages, or not hearing at all in a world of verbal communicative exchanges can result in problems for both the adult with impaired hearing and for those with whom she or he associates who do not possess impaired hearing. For the audiologist, helping people to deal with the problems that are inherent in breakdowns in communication as a result of impaired hearing is an integral part of the process of aural rehabilitation.

OLDER ADULTS WHO POSSESS "IMPAIRED HEARING"

Adults who are considered to be "hearing impaired" are those who possess a hearing loss of various degrees and configurations, but who possess hearing that is to varying degrees probably usable for purposes of communication, although with some difficulty. These persons range from those who require amplification through the use of hearing aids to assist them in hearing speech, to those who possess a milder loss of hearing that requires relatively simple changes in their listening environment for purposes of communication with others.

Hearing impairment among this population of adults can result in breakdowns in communication that can impact negatively on their social and personal lives that can result in depression and withdrawal from situations that require communication. The tendency to withdraw from situations and environments that otherwise involve interactive communication, in turn, can result in personal and social problems that can impact on those important aspects of their lives that, in turn, can have psychological implications.

Counseling provides adults who possess impaired hearing with access to avenues of services that can assist him or her to learn to cope more efficiently within various aspects of their communicative life in spite of their hearing loss, and an understanding of the causes for the difficulties that are being experienced in hearing and communication. With a better understanding of why the difficulties are being experiences, strategies for overcoming them can be developed.

Hearing loss can result in an extremely frustrating disability in interactive verbal communication, which, in turn, can result in other impairments within environments that require communication. Those include one's social life and one's personal life. The adjustments that are required can appear overwhelming to an adult who has never had to consider those adjustments before, and did not expect to. These individuals require special services that are different from those that are offered adults who are "deaf" as described above, and require different strategies for learning to cope in spite of their hearing loss.

DEPRESSION—FEELINGS OF INADEQUACY

People with impaired hearing may feel shut off from the world, not only because of difficulty communicating with others, but also because some or all of the subliminal auditory clues that permit one to maintain contact with the "hearing world" are no longer available. This phenomenon described by Ramsdell (1978) is discussed below. Reaction to this depression may be by withdrawing from social situations and from contact with other people. This might be considered a normal response to an acquired condition rather than a typical reaction of someone who is born deaf and into the unique Culture of Deafness. Depression is frequently complicated by feelings of inadequacy. People who become deaf and even those who become hard of hearing may feel that they should be able to cope better with a hearing loss and that the inability to do so indicates weakness. In addition, there may be feelings of shame, because of the rationalization that hearing difficulty is associated with abnormalities such as thinking, learning, remembering, or decision-making disabilities. They may apologize for not understanding and assume that the "fault" for communication breakdown is always theirs.

DEFENSE MECHANISMS

Denial

In general, threats to self-esteem are handled by one or more defense mechanisms. A common defense mechanism is denial. People with mild to moderate hearing losses may simply not acknowledge they have a hearing loss because to them acceptance implies abnormality. The same individuals would probably have no difficulty accepting the reality of a vision problem, because visual problems tend not to be associated with the general adequacy of the person. Denial increases the problem because it makes it more difficult to seek help or accept the need for a hearing aid because the visibility of the hearing aid would make the hearing impairment apparent to others. It is also a common reaction for the sufferer to assume their communication problems would resolve, if only people would speak plainly.

Hostility and Suspicion

It may be natural again for those who suffer a hearing 'loss" to blame others for their difficulties, accusing them of mumbling or of deliberately excluding them from a conversation. They may become suspicious, accusing others of saying unpleasant things or planning unpleasant situations. Laughter may be misinterpreted as ridicule. They may react negatively to such service providers as a doctor, an audiologist, or a hearing aid dispenser.

The service provider may be the messenger of the bad news and blaming the messenger is common.

It is important for the service provider to be aware of the devastating nature of the message they have the power to convey. Discussing an older patient's hearing loss by dismissing it as something that happens when we get old is of little assurance or assistance to the person receiving this information. Although the patient may admit to suspecting hearing loss it may be no less traumatic than someone who might suspect cancer or terminal illness. Verifying the suspicion, in fact, may be a devastating blow that is internalized along with a polite chuckle to acknowledge the "getting older" comment. It is vital for the service provider to follow up with the patient immediately and frequently. A call to the patient at home the evening of the visit when the hearing loss was determined will be important to the patient. Discussing something that will make life easier under the circumstances such as a headset or wireless assistive device for the TV, may help to sort out the inconvenience of the "loss." As follow-up continues, strategies for coping may be introduced along with support groups, online services, broader assistive technology, and even communication alternatives. The audiologist is notoriously "the demon" with the Deaf as well as those who lose their hearing. The physician makes the actual diagnosis and so should be classified as "co-demon," but typically this is not the case. The reason is simple: the physician calls the patient at home after the visit. Audiologists usually do not do this. The follow-up call to the patient's home and "after hours" is considered a sign of compassion, outreach and understanding and unrelated to the "business of hearing" which is conducted during the workday.

Also, it is vital for the service provider to make some effort to communicate visually or manually with Deaf clientele. Learning to fingerspell requires an evening of effort that can demonstrate to the member of the ASL-based culture that you not only acknowledge the linguistic system but also support the Culture in general. Learning a few signs will go a long way to forming a bond with the Deaf patient. It can instill a sense of trust and help cement the doctor-patient relationship.

PSYCHOLOGICAL LEVELS OF HEARING

Ramsdell (1978) in his classic treatise on hearing loss has described three psychological levels of hearing for the normal hearing person and the problems associated with loss of hearing at each level.

Primitive Level

At the primitive level, sound functions as auditory coupling to the world. Individuals react to the changing background sounds of the world without being aware of it. As Ramsdell (1978) states:

> At this level, we react to such sounds as the tick of a clock, the distant roar of traffic, vague echoes of people moving in other rooms of the house, without being aware that we are hearing them. These incidental noises maintain our feeling of being part of a living world and contribute to our own sense of being alive. (p. 501)

When this primitive function is lost, acute depression may occur. Because the primitive level of hearing is not on a conscious level, the person who is deaf may not be aware of the cause of the depression. Frequently, the depression is attributed to inadequacy in coping with the hearing impairment.

The severity of the depression will be greatest among persons who have a sudden hearing loss, whether it is through trauma, surgery such as acoustic tumor removal, or other causes. Fortunately, hearing loss of sudden onset most frequently affects one ear only, although bilateral losses do occur.

Depression due to the loss of the primitive level will occur in the individual with slowly deteriorating hearing as well. In this case it is more insidious, occurring more slowly, but the resulting depression may be equally great. In some instances, the depression may be more severe because the person may not be aware that hearing is deteriorating. Informing the patient of the true cause of the depression will help alleviate some of the problem, although this knowledge will not eliminate it entirely. Often, properly fitted amplification (hearings aids or cochlear implants) can restore the primitive level, even if speech understanding is not possible. In some cases if amplification is not possible, such as with cranial nerve (CN) VIII destruction, a vibrotactile device may serve to couple the deaf individual to the world of sound.

The loss of the primitive level is a problem primarily with severe to profound adventitious losses. Most adults who are culturally deaf have never experienced the world of sound and, therefore, are not aware of the absence of subliminal auditory cues.

Warning or Signal Level of Hearing

At the warning level, sounds convey information about objects or events. The doorbell indicates the presence of a visitor. Footsteps indicate that someone is approaching. A siren indicates an emergency vehicle is near. A fire alarm indicates danger. Because warning sounds are frequently intense, loss of the warning level is generally found among persons with severe to profound losses. Some warning sounds, however, are of low intensity, and may be missed by persons with less severe hearing losses. These are mainly distant sounds, such as the whistle of an approaching train.

Psychological Impact of Hearing Loss

Insecurity

When the ability to hear warning sounds such as a smoke alarm, a door knock, or a child in another room is lost, feelings of insecurity are understandable. Such problems are found within all segments of the deaf and severely hard-of-hearing population, but to a much lesser extent among people who are culturally Deaf. A vast array of electronic visual systems have been developed to deal with warning level problems. These systems can monitor a doorbell, a person in another room, a smoke alarm, and any other important sound within the home or office. More complete discussions of alerting device systems can be found in Compton (1993), DiPietro, Williams, and Kaplan (1984), and Kaplan (1987).

Annoyance

Feelings of annoyance are caused by disruption of normal patterns of life due to loss of hearing at the warning level. The person who is deaf or hard of hearing who cannot hear the alarm clock may oversleep in the morning and suffer penalties at work as a result. When the ring of the telephone can no longer be heard, social activities may be affected or business opportunities lost. Visual alerting systems can be very useful in overcoming these problems.

Localization

Localization problems may be considered a special type of warning level difficulty. To predict direction of sound, approximately equal sensitivity is needed in both ears; therefore, the inability to localize sound is a special problem for persons with unilateral losses. What is not always realized, however, is that localization problems also exist for individuals who have bilateral hearing impairment who are aided monaurally.

In addition to alerting device technology, warning level difficulties can be dealt with by training a person who is hard-of-hearing or deaf to become more visually aware of his or her environment.

Loss of Esthetic Experiences

For many individuals, music provides an esthetic experience. For some people the inability to hear the sounds of nature, such as bird calls, may represent significant esthetic loss. Amplification cannot always restore these sounds to the extent that esthetic experiences are restored.

Symbolic Level of Hearing

At the symbolic level, individuals deal with sound as language and a major channel of communication. Nearly all people who are deaf or hard-of-hearing have difficulty at this level to one degree or another. Many children and adults who have deafness early in childhood experience delayed English language development, which later affects reading and other academic skills. Although adults who are culturally Deaf tend to communicate comfortably in sign language and consider English a second language, they may have difficulties with the vocabulary and structure of English. English language deficits create a variety of communication problems for anyone who needs to function within the mainstream community for any reason.

Although adults who are hard-of-hearing or deafened generally do not suffer delayed language development, they do face the problem of communicating under conditions of reduced verbal redundancy imposed by impaired auditory reception. Depending on degree, type, and configuration of loss, such individuals lose linguistic cues inherent in a sentence, prosodic cues such as stress and inflection, and phonemic information. The fewer auditory cues that are available, the more likely a person is to misinterpret what is heard, with consequent embarrassment, frustration, and social penalty. This situation is worsened if the communication environment has background noise, competing speech, or other auditory or visual distractions.

At Home

The home can be a source of tension because of communication difficulties for a number of reasons. First, there is more opportunity for interpersonal communication and, consequently, more opportunity for communication breakdown. Second, the person who is hard-of-hearing or deaf expects the family to be more understanding of the special problems imposed by hearing loss than nonrelatives and is disappointed if that is not the case. Third, households tend to be noisy places. The noise level in a typical kitchen was measured at 100 dB SPL with water running at moderate speed, the refrigerator on, and the radio tuned to a comfortable listening level. Competing noise may give the hard of hearing person no usable hearing whatsoever. This fact is puzzling especially to children in the family who may not fully appreciate how the hearing loss can seem so selective. How is it that conversation can be at a normal level and without misunderstandings in the quiet living room and yet be impossible in the kitchen? The strain of hearing may be too great when the sufferer is exhausted at the end of the day. What comes naturally to the family members requires concentration and oftentimes great effort by the person with hearing loss. Sorting through a mental catalog of likely utterances that were made in the context leaves the sufferer mentally and physically challenged at the end of a day of this endless activity.

When there are pre-existing conflicts already within a family, a hearing loss can accentuate them. The hearing impairment can be used as a weapon either by the person who is hard-of-hearing or by other family members. A supportive family is important to an individual who is deaf or hard-of-hearing; at the same time, the person with the hearing loss must be willing to assume part of the responsibility for successful communication.

An individual who is culturally Deaf will not have communication difficulties with the family, if the family is willing and able to use sign language as the primary mode of communication. However, the majority of adults who are culturally Deaf grew up in hearing families. Unless the deaf person can communicate orally with the family or the family can sign to the deaf person, limited communication occurs in the home and the stresses are great.

The Telephone

A special problem at the symbolic level is inability to use the telephone. The telephone message has become an integral part of our lives, affecting communication at home, work, school, and in social environments. The person who cannot understand speech transmitted by telephone or who cannot hear the telephone ring is affected in every aspect of life. Social contacts are reduced because friends and family cannot be easily contacted. Vocational opportunities are limited to the minority of jobs not requiring telephone use. The inability to use the telephone to summon help is threatening, particularly for an individual who lives alone. However, many of these inconveniences are overcome with text-message capability and E-mail. In fact, the majority of young adults with normal hearing may prefer this communication method generally, and Deaf young adults use it constantly.

Many people who are deaf or hard-of-hearing can learn to use the telephone more effectively by developing appropriate telephone strategies. Telecommunication devices for the deaf (TDDs) are viable options for those who cannot use the voice telephone and video phone technology is available to all deaf and hard-of-hearing persons.

Social Activities

For many adults, sudden or increasing hearing loss results in a restriction of social activities. The difficulty in understanding speech exposes individuals who are deaf or hard-of-hearing to the danger and embarrassment of misinterpreting what is said. As a result, they may react inappropriately and be exposed to ridicule. It is a rare person who possesses enough ego strength to continually explain the presence of a hearing loss and continually ask people to repeat what has been said. Even well-meaning friends do not always succeed in making a person who is deaf or hard-of-hearing feel comfortable.

People with normal hearing may feel uncomfortable when they know a listener does not understand what is being said. Often they are at a loss as to how to help the listener understand better, particularly when the person who is deaf or hard-of-hearing attempts to "bluff" and does it badly. Both partners in the conversation may attempt to deny a hearing loss, but communication is disrupted and speaker and listener are embarrassed.

When the hearing loss is severe or has been present for a long time, speech may deteriorate. In that case, the person who is deaf or hard-of-hearing may not be clearly understood, adding to the possible social penalties imposed by the hearing loss.

Conversational difficulties increase exponentially in difficult listening situations. Following a conversation alternating between members of a group can be very difficult, particularly with background noise. A dinner party can be extremely anxiety-provoking and a cocktail party impossible.

Social activities are further limited when a person who is deaf or hard-of-hearing can no longer enjoy the theater or lectures. Just as in face-to-face conversation, the person must cope with speakers or actors who may not project adequately, speech that shifts rapidly from one person to another, and poor room acoustics, as well as the loss of sensitivity and distortion imposed by the hearing loss.

More and more, as social activities become restricted, the person who is deaf or hard-of-hearing is isolated and lonely. This condition may ultimately be accepted with resignation, or it may be met with aggression. The individual may deny the reality of the problem and attribute a shrinking social life to the malice of others. Regardless of whether the problem is met with resignation or aggression, the person who is deaf or hard-of-hearing suffers deterioration in the quality of his or her lifestyle.

Individuals who are culturally Deaf do not suffer social penalties because of hearing loss so long as their social contacts remain within the Deaf community. That is usually a satisfying and enriching social choice. However, those who wish to socialize outside of the Deaf culture encounter the same barriers as individuals who are hard-of-hearing and individuals who are not culturally Deaf. Generally, successful cross-cultural friendships occur when a hearing person can sign comfortably and both parties are good communicators.

Other Problems at the Symbolic Level

Every person who is deaf or hard-of-hearing has had, at one time or another, difficulties in obtaining services. This may involve mailing a package at the post office, purchasing an airline ticket, placing an order at a restaurant, or communicating effectively with a physician. Persons who are deaf or hard-of-hearing are at a definite disadvantage when dealing with the law. In recognition of this, a legal center for the Deaf was established at Gallaudet University. Most hospitals attempt to make special provisions for communicating with patients who are deaf or hard-of-hearing, but personnel are not always aware of their communication problems. Hearing aids may be removed for safekeeping, effectively destroying any possible communication.

Another problem at the symbolic level is the ability to hear and understand television. Many people who are hard-of-hearing increase the volume beyond the tolerance level of hearing family members and neighbors, thereby creating a great deal of tension. Many people who are deaf cannot understand the TV signal, regardless of its intensity. The inability to enjoy television is not only a social loss, but eliminates an important source of information. Assistive device technology can make television accessible to almost everyone (Compton, 1993). In addition, many people who are deaf or hard-of-hearing find the use of closed captioning very useful.

FACILITATING ADJUSTMENT

The professional faces a twofold task in helping the person who is deaf or hard-of-hearing adjust to the problems imposed by hearing impairment. First, through educational and personal adjustment counseling (Sanders, 1988), patients must be helped to accept themselves as people who are deaf or hard-of-hearing and understand the limitations imposed by the hearing loss. Once this is achieved, patients can be helped to manipulate the environment to minimize penalties. Environmental manipulation may involve use of listening aids, modification of communication situations, and education of family, friends, and associates.

DEFINITION OF THE PROBLEM

To provide meaningful assistance to a patient who is hard-of-hearing or deaf, it is necessary to obtain information on the specific communicative difficulties encountered in daily activities. Not only is it important to identify specific difficult listening situations, but also to assess coping strategies and attitudes of a patient toward communication and toward him- or herself as a person with a hearing loss.

To one degree or another, the traditional case history explores areas of communicative difficulty and allows the interviewer to assess an individual's motivation to cope with communicative difficulties. However, a case history interview provides only a general overview of a patient's communicative difficulties. It does not provide quantitative information about degree of difficulty in various situations, nor generally does it sufficiently and systematically probe the specific social, vocational, and interpersonal situations creating problems. There are a number of communication scales available to provide more precise evaluation about difficult communication situations, communication strategies used by the patient, and attitudes about hearing loss. This information helps an aural rehabilitation specialist to plan a program of therapy and observe progress as it occurs.

COUNSELING

The Process

After the specific communicative and attitudinal problems of a patient have been defined, a specific aural rehabilitation program needs to be developed to meet the identified needs. In addition to speechreading, auditory training, and other skill development activities, personal adjustment and informational counseling must be included in the program as needed.

Personal Adjustment Counseling

Although personal adjustment and informational counseling are artificially separated here for purposes of discussion, they are intertwined in an actual rehabilitative program. The personal adjustment counselor functions as a facilitator to help patients modify maladaptive attitudes about themselves as hearing-impaired persons. Kodman (1967) discusses three facilitative conditions that must be present, if the therapist is to be successful.

Accurate Empathy

The first condition is accurate empathy. This is the understanding by a therapist of the true feelings that underlie statements the patient might make. The therapist then responds in such a way that the patient's feelings are reflected back, so that his or her difficulties can be viewed objectively. For example, a patient might say, "Most people don't speak plainly these days. I'd rather read a book than talk to people." The empathetic clinician might reply, "It must be terribly frustrating not to understand people. Let's talk about some of your experiences." As the patient begins to relate difficult listening experiences, the therapist can continue reflecting back upon the patient's feelings and perhaps, in the process, lead the patient to suggest ways of coping with these situations. This is a nondirective approach. The patient makes decisions based on increased perception of the situation; decisions are not imposed on the patient.

The use of accurate empathy is as important in a group situation as in an individual session. In the group situation, the therapist must reflect the feelings of each member as they are expressed. After a group becomes a cohesive unit, the members may begin to practice accurate empathy toward each other, providing strong positive reinforcement for attitudinal change.

Unconditional Positive Regard

The second condition is unconditional positive regard. This involves acceptance of patients as they are, regardless of any hostility, belligerence, or apparent lack of cooperation. It is sometimes difficult for a novice clinician to accept expressions of negativism from a patient and not to consider such behavior as a personal attack. However, it is important to realize that unpleasant actions or expressions are simply manifestations of a patient's problems. Perspective taking, the ability to take another's point of view (Erdmann, 1993), is a combination of accurate empathy and unconditional positive regard. Patient management is facilitated if an aural rehabilitation specialist can view experiences from the patient's point of view.

Genuineness

A third facilitative condition is genuineness. This condition implies a relaxed, friendly attitude toward a patient, respect for the patient's suggestions, ability to accept criticism, and communication with the patient in a manner he or she can easily understand. A genuine clinician does not retreat into professional jargon or assume a pose of superiority because of professional stature.

These facilitative conditions are especially important when working with patients who are culturally deaf. Their language and culture must be understood and respected. American Sign Language (ASL) is not English; idioms and other figurative language vary from English. ASL tends to be a more direct language, with different pragmatic conventions and far fewer euphemisms than English; expression of ideas tends to be more direct. What may appear to be rudeness may simply reflect differences in the languages. To work effectively with a person who is culturally Deaf, it is important for a clinician to have a working knowledge of the patient's language and be willing to use it. Even if the clinician is not fluent in ASL, he or she should make every effort to maximize communication with the patient. Most people who are culturally deaf will meet hearing clinicians half way communicatively, if convinced of the genuineness of the relationship.

Patients who are culturally Deaf sometimes make decisions from a different cultural base than patients who are not culturally deaf or are hard-of-hearing. Some have no desire to mainstream into majority culture; these people enter into therapy with a desire to develop greater communicative independence in those situations where it is advantageous to communicate using English speech or writing. The aural rehabilitation specialist must respect such decisions and work with patients on their own terms.

The qualities of accurate empathy, unconditional positive regard, and genuineness can be developed or enhanced through experience. Audio- or videotaping sessions, with the permission of the patient, of course, and later reviewing the patient-clinician interchange is an excellent way for the novice clinician to improve skills.

Accepting the Reality of the Hearing Loss

One of the most important goals of personal adjustment counseling is to help a patient accept the reality of the hearing loss and the need for help. One must not assume that because a patient has opted for a clinic evaluation, that acceptance of amplification or therapy is a given. The patient may simply be appeasing family or friends or perhaps be taking the first tenuous steps toward seeking help although remaining ambivalent about self-acceptance as a hard-of-hearing person. There is no point in recommending amplification if a patient is not ready to accept it.

It is far better to persuade the individual to enroll in an aural rehabilitation program that includes discussion-counseling to help with acceptance of the reality of the hearing problem. If necessary, the group discussions can be supplemented with individual counseling. It must be made clear that participation in aural rehabilitation is not contingent on hearing aid use. It must be emphasized that the audiologist is ready to assist with selection of a hearing aid if and when a patient becomes ready.

Recognizing a Patient's Fears

When a person feels a loss of self-esteem because of an inability to hear normally, he or she has a tendency to conceal the hearing loss. The fear is often related to the concern that people will view him or her as different. To such an individual, a hearing aid is a visible indication that he or she is an inferior person. Although it may be recognized logically that there is no truth to such fears, a fearful person may not be able to emotionally accept use of a hearing aid. Even when the hearing aid can be completely hidden from view, the problem of acceptance is not solved for some people; they believe that wearing a hearing aid represents tangible evidence of inferiority. These feelings are especially prevalent among adolescents, where peer identification and acceptance are overriding concerns. In addition, many adolescents and adults fear that hearing loss and its visible badge, the hearing aid, will make them less attractive to the opposite sex.

If an individual who is deaf or hard-of-hearing does succeed in working through the emotional objections to amplification, the usual expectation is that the hearing aid will restore good hearing. If the hearing aid user is not properly prepared for the limitations of amplification and the adjustment necessary to use it well, he or she will be disappointed during attempts to use the hearing aid. If the hearing aid is discarded, the person who is deaf or hard-of-hearing may feel even more isolated and depressed, as hopes of solving his or her communication problem with a mechanical prosthesis have not been fulfilled.

Educational, or Informational, Counseling

Educational or informational counseling is the provision of information about hearing loss, its effect on communication, and intervention procedures. Although this type of counseling can be accomplished either in an individual or a group situation, the group situation is often more effective, because experiences can be shared and peer reinforcement can occur. However, group participation requires that individuals identify themselves as persons with hearing problems. If a patient is not ready for this level of acceptance, individual therapy is preferable until the goal of ultimate participation in a group can be met.

Topics that should be included in an informational counseling program are:

- The nature of the auditory system and hearing loss, including interpretation of audiograms.

- Effects of hearing loss on communication and impact of background noise and poor listening conditions.

- Importance of visual input, audiovisual integration, and attending behavior.

- Impact of talker differences and social conditions to communication.

- Benefits and limitations of speechreading.

- Benefits and limitations of hearing aids and their use and care.

- Benefits and limitations of assistive devices.

- Use of community resources such as self-help groups.

Identifying Difficult Listening Situations

An important part of informational counseling is identification of difficult communication situations and development of coping strategies that work. The group format is especially effective for identification of and practice with communication strategies, but such training can be incorporated into individual sessions, if necessary.

Assertiveness Training

Assertiveness training easily can be incorporated into aural rehabilitation sessions. It is important for patients who are deaf or hard-of-hearing to understand that they have a right to understand, that it is acceptable to ask for help in a polite, courteous fashion, and that it is the responsibility of the person with hearing loss to instruct the communication partner in ways of helping. Patients need to learn to distinguish between: (1) aggressive, which involves violation of other people's rights; (2) passive, which involves allowing others to violate their rights; and (3) assertive, in which patients protect their rights without violating those of other people.

The aural rehabilitation specialist might pose the problem: "Suppose you meet two friends on a noisy street who are having a conversation. They greet you and try to include you in their conversation, but you are unable to follow what they are saying. What might you do?" The therapist would then try to elicit some of the following examples of assertive behavior:

1. Ask the people to move away from the source of the noise so that you can understand better.

2. Ask one of the two people to briefly summarize what has been said before you entered the conversation.

3. Admit you do not understand and ask for repetition or rephrasing of an idea.

4. Ask the people to speak louder.

The patients would then be asked to give examples of aggressive behavior, such as verbal or physical abuse of the speakers, and of passive behavior, such as saying nothing about the lack of understanding.

Role-playing can be incorporated into assertiveness training sessions very effectively to help patients define appropriate behaviors. Homework assignments involving the use of these behaviors in actual life situations can follow the role playing and be followed up by discussions during subsequent classes.

Once patients are able to function assertively, they are ready to learn the many behaviors that facilitate communication. Among the most effective communication strategies are those that involve "anticipation."

Strategies Involving Anticipation

Strategies involving anticipation, sometimes called "Anticipatory Strategies," include thinking about a communication situation in advance and figuring out ways to minimize difficulties. They include such things as educating speakers to keep their faces visible, coming early to a meeting to get a seat close to the speaker, identifying tables in restaurants that provide optimal lighting and minimal noise, and making advance reservations to secure those tables, arranging for note-takers or interpreters in classes or meetings, and obtaining assistive devices. An excellent anticipatory strategy involves predicting vocabulary or dialogue that is likely to occur in a particular situation and practicing such language in advance. Patients need to learn how to use such strategies and when they are appropriate. Detailed discussion of communication strategies and exercises for practice can be found in Kaplan, Bally, and Garretson (1987), Tye-Murray (1991, 1993), and Tye-Murray, Purdy, and Woodworth (1992).

It is important to realize that it is difficult for many people who deaf or hard-of-hearing to be assertive, particularly as they are often rebuffed. Coping with difficult listening situations in the manner suggested requires practice and development of a "thick skin." Clinicians should be sure to make their patients understand that they are aware of the difficulties involved in implementing these suggestions.

Educating Significant Others

Because communication involves not only the person who is deaf or hard-of-hearing but also family members, friends, and others, educational counseling of these people is important to the adjustment of the patient. Family members or associates must understand the nature of a patient's hearing problem and the specific ways in which communication is affected. After testing it is highly desirable to include spouses, children, parents, or friends in the counseling session for the initial explanation of the hearing loss.

The limitations imposed by some types of hearing loss are baffling to the lay person who finds it difficult to understand why some things can be heard easily and other conversations are handled poorly. The effect of a high-frequency hearing loss on speech perception, the practical effects of a word recognition problem, and the devastating effects of competing noise or competing speech on speech understanding must be carefully explained. For complete understanding, several explanations at different times may be necessary for both a patient and significant others. For that reason, normal-hearing family members or friends should be encouraged to enter a rehabilitation group with a patient.

SUMMARY

The psychological impact of hearing impairment or deafness on adults is real and can be severe. The avenues available to those who serve these persons can be employed in constructive and meaningful ways to restore feelings of self-worth and to assist patients in adjusting to the demands of their world. Only audiologists who are willing to enter into a close working relationship with these adults with hearing impairment should become a part of the process of facilitative counseling.

CHAPTER 4

Special Considerations for the Use of Hearing Aids for Older Adults

This chapter focuses on how amplification can be considered as part of the program to support older adults who posses impaired hearing. The fitting and dispensing of hearing aids and other amplification systems and devices are important aspects of the process of rehabilitation on behalf of hearing-impaired older adults. When an older adult's level of auditory acuity is brought to a more efficient level through the appropriate fitting of a hearing aid, then other components of a program of support are facilitated. For many older individuals, a properly fitted and properly used hearing aid will enhance their ability to interact more competently and more enjoyably in their social, personal, and economic life.

FACTORS INFLUENCING SUCCESSFUL HEARING AID USE BY OLDER ADULTS

As discussed in Chapter 1, hearing loss and accompanying auditory impairment found among many older adults is quite complex. In older individuals who possess both a sensorineural hearing loss and a compounding central auditory impairment, a hearing aid per se may not resolve all of the hearing problems being experienced by the person (Humes, 2008; Rawool, 2007; Stach, 1990). Hull (1998, 2001a, 2009) discussed the additive factors that older persons experience when attempting to understand speech through a peripheral and central auditory system that is no longer programmed for the speed and agility required for comprehending rapid adult speech, and that must also cope with less than beneficial environmental/listening conditions along with imprecise speakers. In other words, it is important to consider the possibility that a hearing aid candidate's hearing test results may not reveal all that is important when recommending the individual for a hearing aid fitting, as CNS auditory involvement and external factors can negatively influence performance in speech comprehension with and without amplification.

In an early treatise on hearing aid considerations for elderly adults, Kasten (1981) stated that there are nine important factors that go beyond a person's auditory function that must be considered when determining the appropriateness of amplification for older adults. Those are: (1) their motivation, (2) their adaptability, (3) their personal appraisal, (4) money, (5) their social context, (6) personal influences, (7) mobility, (8) vanity, and (9) manual dexterity.

Motivation

In their early writings, Rupp, Higgins, and Maurer (1977) consider *motivation* as being the most important factor in their feasibility scale for predicting successful hearing aid use. They point out that those who show less personal motivation and depend more on the urging of others to procure a hearing aid are less likely to be successful in the use of amplification. Likewise, the individual who has a great desire to continue to lead a mentally, physically, and emotionally active life and to participate in the affairs of society is more likely to be a successful user of hearing aids. On the other hand, those who have lost interest in their surroundings and are willing to withdraw from society may have little motivation or desire to be successful in the use of amplification. Thus, the probability of these persons being successfully rehabilitated through hearing aid use becomes correspondingly less.

Adaptability

New hearing aid users are sometimes quite surprised when they first experience amplification. It is likely that some people expect a hearing aid to restore their hearing to the efficiency that it had in previous years, whereas others may expect it to be nothing but a nuisance. It is almost certain that neither of these expectations are realistic or correct. If an individual expects essentially complete correction of the hearing deficiency, he or she will almost certainly be disappointed. Conversely, if an individual has so little optimism as to think that the hearing aid will be of no help, then he or she may be unwilling to put forth the effort that is necessary to become oriented to and consequently wear the instruments. In other words, the person simply may be unwilling to give amplification a chance. If a person is unwilling to try something new or unusual, then major changes in attitude are probably necessary before successful hearing aid use will be noted.

Personal Appraisal

An individual's personal assessment and emotional feelings about his or her communication problems are extremely important factors in the degree of success expected from amplification. In other words, audiological assessment data are appropriate in determining the degree of hearing loss, but self-assessment regarding its effect on their ability to function communicatively is also important.

Successful use of amplification is most likely when there is a positive correlation between the two sets of information, audiometric data and self-assessment. One who is able to appraise his or her personal disability objectively and with accuracy generally is in a position to at least accept the resulting communication problems and assist in developing a realistic approach to the possibilities for improvement, as well as to the specific procedures needed to overcome the negative impact of the hearing loss to the degree possible.

Money

The financial status of a person can certainly have a profound effect on his or her willingness to use hearing aids. For the majority of potential users, however, the purchase of hearing aids is not impossible. On the other hand, hearing aids still may be in the category of a luxury and would probably be purchased only if the person who has hearing impairment is convinced that they will meet his or her needs on an absolute basis. Many people are aware that their friends and, perhaps they themselves, may have spent thousands of dollars for one or more hearing aids that proved to be unsatisfactory and were relegated to a dresser drawer or closet shelf after the return warranty ran out. Thus, some people are unwilling to spend the money necessary to obtain hearing aids. When an individual is living on a fixed income and is only meeting living expenses, then the matter of hearing aid purchase may become financially difficult.

Those who are eligible for Medicaid assistance can sometimes obtain help from that source to purchase hearing aids (if their state Medicaid laws provide for hearing aids). However, some states (e.g., California, Kansas, and others) only provide one hearing aid every 3 to 5 years unless the patient has other special circumstances such as blindness. Hearing aid banks can be an important resource and there may be other possibilities for financial assistance by civic organizations. However, these sources also may have restrictions that present problems in carrying out a purchase.

Social Context

The older patient who has hearing impairment, as any other person, may fit anywhere along a continuum from one who is socially active to one who is socially isolated. Those who are active in various aspects of social life are ones who are likely to desire to maintain contact with other people and to communicate actively. Those who are isolated, either self-imposed or geographically, on the other hand, may have lost interest in such contact. Thus, it becomes the task of the audiologist to determine if their withdrawal from social contact is due to hearing loss, or due to other reasons.

It seems reasonable to assume that those who are engaged in social activities would be most likely to be successful in rehabilitation utilizing hearing aids. At least they would have the desire and motivation for that type of achievement. Conversely, those who are withdrawn or who lack social awareness might be the ones least likely to be successful in rehabilitation utilizing hearing aids.

The large remaining group includes those who are neither extremely active socially nor completely withdrawn. They are, in fact, the ones who are in the process of losing their interest in social contact because too great an effort is needed to maintain communication with their friends or colleagues. Although their lagging interest in social affairs would make them less than ideal candidates for the use of amplification, it is also highly likely that satisfactory selection of amplification and the use of appropriate rehabilitation procedures can improve the probability of re-entry into social activities.

Personal/Functional Influences

The attitudes, interests, and activities of the friends and family of the older person who has hearing impairment can have a great deal of influence on his or her attitudes and desires. If the person is still employed or active in volunteer or avocational activities that involve him or her with communication and, if the people who are associated with the person who has hearing impairment are sympathetic, understanding, and stimulating in their conversations, then the elderly person's desire to utilize amplification will be enhanced. Conversely, if the living situation and the people involved in the life process of the older person lack stimulating ingredients, then the individual who has hearing impairment is likely to have little reason for wanting to try to obtain or adjust to the use of amplification.

Mobility

Restrictions in physical mobility can have an impact on older adults and their willingness to use hearing aids and other prosthetic devices. For example, if an individual is mobile and able to be involved in various activities including church, theater, musical concerts, and favorite social clubs, then he or she is likely to be a good candidate for the use of amplification and improved communication. On the other hand, those who are limited in mobility and who rarely leave their immediate vicinity for social or business contacts may have less apparent need for communication and, therefore, less need and/or desire for amplification. Furthermore, there are those who desire to live alone and may have little desire for communication with others. They may feel a great deal of loneliness, yet they are unable or unwilling to make the effort to maintain contact with other people.

These persons may have a need for the communicative assistance that can be obtained through amplification, yet they often are physically and emotionally limited in their ability and/or desire to become involved in social activities, and, thus, their ability or desire to utilize amplification. They might have other types of debilitating impairments in addition to the hearing impairment, yet they may be able to participate in social activities, for example, if transportation was available. However, the hearing problem presents an additional barrier, and the combination of impairments results in greater isolation. The result is that they may be less successful from the standpoint of improvements in social contact and their ability to communicate than we as rehabilitation specialists expect them to be. However, the lack of improvements in hearing and communication may be from default rather than from their desire to isolate themselves.

Vanity

Vanity is an aspect of human nature that can have a great impact on a person's interest in trying to adjust to hearing aids. Corrective lenses for the eyes is an example of how a prosthetic appliance can be widely accepted. Many people would prefer not to wear eyeglasses, but, nevertheless, a large majority of our society eventually may need to wear some type of visual correction. In fact, most people accept the use of corrective lenses gracefully at some time in their lives and may even consider it stylish to wear them. Once an individual has accepted the necessity of eyeglasses, he or she may go to extremes by purchasing large and gaudy eyewear, which definitely calls attention to them. On the other hand, based on their own opinions of appearance of self or the opinions of others, persons may try to use contact lenses or corrective surgery to conceal a sight problem as much as possible. Sunglasses are thought of as glamorous and most people, young and old, wear them for both utility to protect their eyes and for style.

Hearing aids have not received the same level of acceptance as eyeglasses. And, it is unlikely that anyone would buy overly large or conspicuous hearing aids in the same way that some people buy large or unusual pairs of eye glasses. On the contrary, most people are interested in being fit with hearing aids that are as small and inconspicuous as possible. A large behind-the-ear instrument is frequently rejected in favor of smaller all-in-the-ear or miniature open-canal models, simply because the person feels that this would be less conspicuous, but still beneficial. Some older persons state strongly that they might accept an in-the-ear instrument, but would not consider a postauricilar aid, even though the latter may provide them better hearing. On the other hand, some people are unwilling to wear an instrument of any kind, because they do not wish to advertise that they have a hearing problem. They would prefer to try to "get by" and try to conceal it. This type of attitude has historically presented a barrier in acceptance of amplification. However, this view appears to be diminishing, as people of the current generation take charge of their own destiny by doing whatever is necessary to reduce barriers to their lives.

Dexterity

Hearing aids and their controls continue to become smaller. This reduction in size has made hearing aids more acceptable to a larger number of people than ever before. For the vast majority of the population, the smaller size has not presented a great problem. However, with advancing age and physical limitations that can accompany aging, the reduction in the dimensions of instruments and the resulting decrease in the size of the controls and batteries can present difficulties. On the other hand, with the advent of programmable instruments, in many cases the only part of the hearing aid that requires manipulation is the battery compartment lid.

With age, the sense of touch may diminish, and people can find it difficult to know precisely if they are correctly seating a hearing aid or earmold into the concha, or if they actually have the battery in place. Elderly adults may be seen with a hearing aid hanging precariously from his or her ear, or with an ear mold that is far from being seated properly. The individual may be unaware about the situation even though he or she has just inserted the hearing aid. These individuals may complain that the hearing aid does not work properly or that it hurts their ear, or that it squeals; both complaints may be easily resolved by ensuring that the aid is properly seated in the ear. Likewise, an older person may have such a poor sense of touch that he or she is unable to find the volume control or the off–on switch. When the person tries to move a control to a desired location, the person may not be certain whether the movement was successful. Even though a specific model of hearing may have internal controls, and all have been preset at the fitting, one must still insert the hearing aid properly in order for it to work as intended.

Thus, good manual dexterity and a good sense of touch can help a great deal in the successful use of amplification. On the other hand, reduced dexterity and sense of touch can be strong deterrents to success, and almost certainly require the assistance of some relative or other person to overcome this difficulty. A mandatory portion of every hearing aid fitting with an older individual should include a dexterity check to determine if the person can use the controls, fit the aids to the ears, and actually handle and change batteries. The fitter should note any problems and consider the need for larger or stacked volume controls, or fitting with internal preset controls, or fitting a programmable instrument that has no external switch or other controls.

CONSIDERATIONS FOR DIFFERENT POPULATIONS OF OLDER ADULTS

There are several populations of older adults who must be considered, and the differences among these populations influence the potential use of hearing aids. The differences among these populations influence the procedures that can be used for selecting a suitable hearing aid.

The Independent Older Adult

Older individuals in the independent group are frequently the easiest to work with and the most successful in terms of hearing aid use. They continue to be in control of their lifestyles and will enter into the process of hearing aid use with their eyes open, although sometimes reluctantly. For the factors or prognostic areas that predict hearing aid use, individuals in this population are most frequently amenable to change. These individuals often continue to be involved in varied activities, and are frequently willing to modify behavior and attitudes for their own betterment.

With the independent-living population, *motivation* is the critical factor. When motivation exists, appropriate counseling can bring about positive change in a patient. Sympathetic support on the part of a spouse or friend can clearly help to strengthen the degree of communicative success.

To a large degree, potential success with hearing aids is directly tied to the extent that a potential hearing aid user can see and experience success in significant and meaningful communication situations. Success in communication can cause a heightened social awareness and can lead to a genuine desire to expand social horizons and to modify an individual's personal life.

The Semi-Independent Older Adult

When clinicians work with the semi-independent population they are faced with a different set of circumstances. These individuals frequently have large portions of their lifestyles dictated by those who control the environment in which they live. In some instances this direction is provided by well-meaning but naive sons or daughters in whose homes the older person may reside; that is, naïve to the special needs of older adults. All too often, this group of older individuals find themselves living in a relatively comfortable, although controlled, environment, and they may think that their only other option is nursing home placement. As a result, their psychological set and their attitude toward the factors relating to successful hearing aid use are consciously or subconsciously dictated to them by the individual or individuals governing their living accommodations.

With this population, it is frequently necessary to spend as much time with the persons who control the living environment as with the older individuals, themselves. If the well-meaning son or daughter is not sold on the value of hearing aids, then the older individual may not be convinced that they will help. If the son or daughter feels that hearing aids are too expensive to warrant purchase, the likelihood is high that the older individual will find no way to afford the purchase. If the son or daughter strongly states that the older person does not seem to have enough of a problem to warrant hearing aid use, then chances are that the older family member will at least verbalize a similar opinion. If the son or daughter feels that the older person does not have a wide enough range of activities or experiences to benefit from a hearing aid, then the likelihood is quite high that the older person will reflect the same belief and, even worse, may demonstrate it.

In spite of the apparent needs of an older individual, then, decisions about amplification and attitudes toward amplification may be shaped by others who are not directly experiencing the problem. On the other hand, family members can also be a catalyst in the successful use of hearing aids.

The former situation creates an awkward position for the older individual who has impaired hearing. He or she may readily recognize the need for the kind of assistance that can be obtained from amplification, but genuinely fear the consequences of a decision that goes contrary to the power structure in his or her environment. Although often not intentional, the older individual in the semi-independent population may become the *recipient* of attitudes and decisions rather than the *originator* of their own attitudes and decisions.

The Dependent Older Adult

The dependent-living population frequently requires a different approach and demands serious moral judgments on the part of the audiologist or other service provider. Individuals in this population may be almost totally controlled and cared for as the result of their physical, emotional, or health condition. If this population is viewed objectively in terms of hearing aid use, clinicians are faced with the fact that they may have poor motivation, little adaptability, limited insight in terms of personal appraisement, little available money, poor social awareness, and a restricted social environment, as well as limited mobility and finger dexterity.

In addition to these factors, we must realize that these people often are cared for by well-meaning and hard-working staff members of health care facilities who know almost nothing about hearing aid use and avenues for communication with adults who posses impaired hearing, and who primarily are concerned with physical factors relating to the maintenance of the patient's daily physical needs. Taken as a group, the prospects for successful hearing aid use are rather limited. Three general attitudes can appear among dependent older individuals who chose not to become involved in hearing aid use: (1) they may deny that a problem is present; (2) they may display a general attitude of hopelessness; and/or (3) they may express recognition of the hearing loss, but may indicate no desire for any type of rehabilitation (Hull, 2009).

Successful Hearing Aid Use for Dependent Older Persons

For dependent older persons, a key to successful hearing aid use may, for example, be staff members who care for the individual or the volunteers who help in activities of daily living. These people must be trained in proper hearing aid use and maintenance and must be schooled on the importance of hearing aids for communication. Through in-services, for example, that explain in detail the methods and procedures they can use to support the older individual who has hearing impairment. They should also receive knowledge about hearing aid use and care.

Clinicians must realize, however, that there generally is a relatively high turnover of staff in many health care facilities. As a rule, the work is hard, the hours are long, and the pay is often not commensurate with the work involved. As a result, many individuals stay with a particular job only until they are able to find something else that will provide them with more satisfaction or more money. With this in mind, clinicians must realize that in-service training that deals with communication strategies and hearing aid use and care must be performed on a recurring basis and must include hands-on demonstration of hearing aid maintenance and use.

With the dependent group, clinicians must remember that well-fitted hearing aids are not an end unto themselves. Hearing aid use will be successful only if there is a need for communication, a desire for personal interaction, and support that includes family and staff encouragement and understanding. Hearing aid use will be successful only when older individuals can demonstrate to themselves a real benefit.

A Final Consideration as It Relates to the Extremely Dependent Older Adult

One final factor is essential to consider when dealing with the extremely dependent aged population. By definition, individuals in this group may be incapable of caring for themselves and require regular attendance by others who provide for their needs. For the hearing aid user within this group, a significant other person must be knowledgeable and proficient in terms of hearing aid use. He or she must be able to ensure that the hearing aids are working properly, the batteries are appropriate and working, the earmolds or hearing aids are inserted properly, and the hearing aids are set as they should be for the individual. Although these do not seem to be overwhelming tasks, they can be major hurdles for an overworked health care facility staff member who has had limited experience with hearing aid use. The audiologist must maintain close contact with health care facility administrators and nursing staff including nurse aides so that they can be available when staff turnover requires a new staff training program. In this way, continuous care for hearing aid users is more readily ensured.

HEARING AID ORIENTATION

The importance of adequate orientation to hearing aid(s) has been stressed throughout this chapter, but a separate discussion of the essential elements of that important aspect of hearing aid fitting and use is important. Orientation to the use of hearing aids is an essential part of the ongoing hearing rehabilitation program. The fitting and dispensing of hearing aids is just the beginning of the process. If a patient is not comfortable with a hearing aid, its uses, benefits, and limitations, it probably will not be successfully utilized by the patient.

There are generally seven important components of a hearing orientation program:

1. An understanding of the function of the component parts and adjustments of hearing aids;

2. Practice in fitting, adjusting, and maintaining the hearing aid;

3. An understanding of the limitations of amplification;

4. Knowledge of why the particular hearing aid was selected for him or her;

5. How to begin using a newly selected hearing aid;

6. How to troubleshoot hearing aid problems; and

7. The legal rights of persons fit with hearing aids.

Depending on the state of health, alertness, and physical ability of the patient, those key elements should guide the hearing aid orientation program. The hearing aid orientation program need not be restricted to a specified time frame. If the patient is part of an ongoing aural rehabilitation program, hearing aid orientation is an integral part. The patient asks questions, receives answers from the audiologist, requests adjustments regarding the fit of the amplification, and, in this regard, receives comprehensive orientation and adjustment service over time.

If the patient is among the dependent population, it becomes critical that his or her family, significant other, or health care facility staff become members of the hearing aid orientation program, as they may be the ones who place the hearing aids on the patient each day.

Patients and their significant other(s) should be provided practical information about the care and maintenance of the hearing aid(s), and their uses. For example:

1. The patient and those who serve the patient should receive general information about hearing aids, what they are, what they do, what they do not do, and the component parts. There is so much misinformation presented in advertisements about hearing aids, that it behooves the audiologist to provide accurate and informative details.

2. Information on adjusting to the hearing aid is critical to the orientation process. This involves practicing placing the hearing aid in one's ear and removing it; what to expect from the hearing aid in noisy or otherwise distracting environments; and how to adjust the aid.

3. The care of one's hearing aid, including the potential harm from water, hair spray, excessive heat, perspiration, and other factors are important parts of the orientation process. Receiving information on cleaning and caring for the hearing aid is as important as learning how to use it.

4. Telephone use with a hearing aid with or without a telecoil should be a part of the orientation process.

5. Information on what causes "whistles and squeals" is also important for patients to receive. This can be a part of the information presented on, "When do hearing aids or earmolds need repair or replacement?"

6. Battery sizes, materials, life expectancy, increasing battery life, and other information about batteries is also critical to the orientation process. There is almost as much misinformation

available to hearing aid users about batteries as there is about hearing aids, themselves.

An effective and efficient hearing aid orientation process is a critically important part of the fitting of hearing aids. The effectiveness of this part of the aural rehabilitation process can enhance or doom the willingness of patients to use their hearing aid(s).

SUMMARY

The older individual who has hearing impairment may belong to one of several different populations who demonstrate a wide range of skills and abilities. Therefore, it is frequently necessary to modify the procedures for selecting and fitting hearing aids to successfully meet each patient's amplification needs.

It matters little which dependency category an aged person may fit into. Each individual presents a unique set of capabilities and/or limitations and those who serve them must be aware of them as they pertain to each individual.

The growing population of older individuals poses a unique challenge to all persons involved in the hearing health care team. The audiologist must be particularly aware that he or she is not dealing with one large homogeneous group of individuals, but rather with several subgroups who have advanced age as a common factor, and their individual level of ability as a distinctive feature.

CHAPTER 5

Techniques for Improving Listening and Communication Skills for Older Adults Who Possess Impaired Hearing

INTRODUCTION

The process of helping older adults to improve their ability to hear and communicate in spite of impaired hearing is as exciting as it is rewarding. To be involved in the recovery of communication skills that previously may have caused an adult to withdraw from his or her communicating world is, indeed, gratifying. Both the patient and service provider can rejoice in the recovery of those skills. Some older patients recover skills that allow them to participate on a social basis once again, at least with a greater degree of efficiency. Others may simply regain the ability to communicate with their family with greater ease. In light of those gains and, perhaps, a step toward a reinstatement of communicative independence, a person who possesses impaired hearing and his or her service provider have reason to rejoice.

Clinicians cannot, under any circumstances, hope to benefit every older person with impaired hearing. But, in attempting to do so, if some are helped who previously had submitted to a self-imposed withdrawal from family and friends because of the embarrassment resulting from responding inappropriately to misunderstood messages, then service providers can be satisfied that their work is worthwhile.

Because older adults who have hearing impairment have experienced normal to near-normal auditory function during their younger years, and because they generally are fully aware of the communicative difficulties they face, it is important that our services address *their* specific communicative needs. In light of confirmation that auditory disorders found in older adults are quite complex, involving both peripheral and central auditory difficulties, approaches to hearing rehabilitation must accommodate both aspects of the disorder. We indeed are serving complex people who possess complex auditory problems.

AN OVERVIEW OF TYPES OF HEARING REHABILITATION TREATMENT

Individual Versus Group Treatment

Individual Treatment

Some individuals will require individual hearing rehabilitation treatment. In instances in which patients are experiencing communicative difficulties that are not conducive to a group therapy environment because of their individual/personal nature, individual sessions are warranted.

For example, a semiretired 75-year-old physician came to this author with a desire for more efficient communication within his office and examination room. The sessions centered on the specific difficulties he was experiencing in that environment, and he did not desire that they be opened up to group sessions.

Another patient's concern was that her granddaughter's wedding was forthcoming, and she felt that she was not going to be able to hear and understand what people were saying while she stood in the reception line. Her request was to receive some hints on how not to embarrass herself and her family by responding inappropriately to what people were saying to her in the reverberant environment of their church fellowship hall. Her rehabilitation program was based on two sessions of problem-solving and supportive/informational counseling. After successfully working through the potential pitfalls of the communicative demands of her granddaughter's wedding, the woman returned to enter group therapy. The sessions held for this woman were rather personal in regard to the difficulties she was anticipating and, in that instance, she felt that they were not conducive to a group therapy environment, at least at that time. So, her desire for individual sessions was fulfilled.

Other circumstances in which individual treatment sessions would be appropriate include:

1. The patient's hearing impairment and concomitant communicative difficulties are so severe that the patient requires concentrated effort to resolve them to the greatest degree possible before entering a group environment;

2. The patient's emotional response to the auditory impairment and the resulting communicative difficulties are such that group involvement, at that particular time, is contraindicated.

Group Treatment

Group hearing rehabilitative treatment, as discussed later in this chapter, can be extremely motivating for many older adults who

are experiencing impaired hearing. Once the problems and difficulties that are specific to individual patients have been resolved
to the degree possible through work on an individual basis,
patients can move into group treatment, if group services are
warranted (Figure 5–1).

Individuals in group treatment find strength in hearing of
others' successes and failures in their own communicative environments. They gain insights through group discussions and
problem-solving into how best to cope in spite of their hearing
impairment. The camaraderie that develops can be rewarding to
group members as their confidence grows in their ability to take
charge of the difficulties that they have been having in their own
communicative worlds.

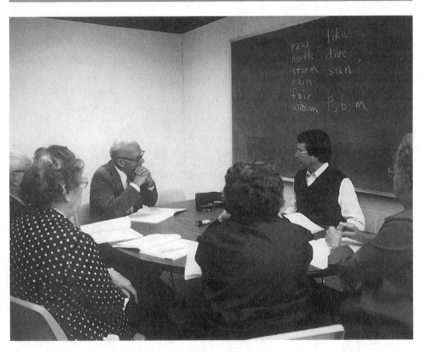

FIGURE 5–1. Group hearing rehabilitation treatment works to allow
patients to share frustrations and triumphs.

COMPONENTS OF
HEARING REHABILITATION TREATMENT

The following are important elements in hearing rehabilitation service programs for older adults that are applicable for either the well adult in the community or those who are confined to a health care facility. They include:

1. Counseling,

2. Hearing aid orientation,

3. Adjusting the listening environment,

4. Development of positive assertiveness,

5. Developing compensatory skills in the use of residual hearing and supplemental visual cues, and

6. Involvement of family and significant others.

Counseling

As this author teaches his students about hearing rehabilitation services for older adults, he emphasizes that counseling, for lack of a better term, is one of the most important aspects and is intertwined throughout the process of hearing rehabilitation. It is not something that occurs alone or out of context. It is an integral part of everything an audiologist does when working with his or her patients. Counseling is called: (1) talking with the patient; (2) instilling confidence in a patient who has become discouraged when he or she did not do as well as expected in a given communicative environment; (3) listening to the feelings a patient reveals about him or herself, or that person's relationship with an intolerant family member or roommate; and (4) trust that must develop between service provider and patient.

Counseling is the *discussion* that develops when a patient desires to talk about an incident in which he or she had particular difficulty understanding what another person was saying. It also includes the *problem-solving* that can unravel the possible reasons for the difficulty, and, one hopes, possible solutions.

This aspect of the process of hearing rehabilitation is, again for lack of a better term, called counseling. But, whatever it is called, it involves *listening, talking, problem-solving, facilitating adjustment* to a frustrating disability, and the *development of trust* between patient and service provider.

When one encounters an older adult with impaired hearing who says, "I do not desire to be helped. I am old and I do not know how much longer I will live," the attitude of the person certainly will influence how much potential progress that he or she will make. This is particularly true if the person has isolated him- or herself from the outside world and is resigned to not seek help because of advanced age.

If there are no other significant contraindicating factors that would hinder responsiveness to hearing rehabilitation services, the audiologist is in a position to serve in a counseling role. It is possible that this person has said what was said because he or she has been told by others that, "You are too old." A well-meaning physician may have said, "You know you're no spring chicken any more." Or, an adult child may have said unthinkingly, "Mom, you know you can't care for yourself as well as you used to, so we should start thinking about moving you to a care facility," not realizing that the older adult is convinced that placement in a "care facility" will be terminal. Such statements, even said in a well-meaning way, are understandably unsettling to an older adult.

One of this author's patients, a woman of 89 years, told me that her 50-year-old daughter told her they should sell her house and she should then move into an efficiency apartment. She was so hurt and angry that she could not think of anything to say. She felt convinced that if her mature daughter felt that she could not care for her house, then she must be doing a worse job than she thought. I asked her what she would have said if her daughter would have suggested that to her when she was 45 years old and her daughter was 15. She said she would have asked her why she would say such a thing, but, she said, "But when you are 89 years old, perhaps it is not worth it."

If the medical records of an individual indicate satisfactory health, and there appears to be nothing that would contraindicate the provision of hearing rehabilitative services, then the self-defeating attitude of the potential patient may be the only thing that stands between the provision of services and reasonable progress in hearing rehabilitation treatment. Although the person's realistic view of becoming older may be a healthy one, long-term mourning because of age and the possibility of death is not. The audiologist can be a positive catalyst in moving beyond aging, particularly for those who are barred from social interaction as a result of their hearing difficulties.

Feelings to Which Service Providers Must Respond

Phrases exemplifying attitudes typical of some older adults who have impaired hearing have been recorded by this author during initial hearing rehabilitation interviews with hundreds of older patients. The feelings that prompted these revealing statements are those that can reduce the desire for hearing rehabilitation services or the progress they may be capable of. They are, furthermore, those to which the audiologist or other service provider must respond. The following are a few of those statements, out of context, recorded by this author as said by some of his patients:

"I feel that I'm on trial, becoming incompetent."

"My son is right behind me. He comes down to see me as often as he can, but he has a lot of business to handle there. I don't see him very often anymore."

I can't hear and my eyes bother me. Surgery won't help my ears or my eyes. I'm told that I'm too old."

"My arthritis bothers me all over, especially with the weather. I used to walk a lot. I can't hear now. I'm too old."

"I fear being alone—being melancholy—with no future to look forward to. I need to find some way to be useful. I can stand a lot. I'm still sturdy."

"I would like, more than anything, to be able to get out, to socialize, but I can't hear very well. I would like to go to church, but the children don't come on Sundays and there is no one to take me."

One statement stands out from all of the rest. It is a statement by a physically strong and mentally alert 82-year-old man who possesses impaired hearing and who is torn between giving up or submitting to the opportunity to improve his ability to function communicatively through an audiologist's services. The statement is, "I'd like to put a younger person on my shoulders to function intellectually on my behalf and hear for me, and to go on from there. But, I suppose I need to learn to rely on myself . . . relationships with people are important, but do I have the potential?"

The above statements are representative of those heard by service providers who accept the opportunity to provide a significant rehabilitative service on behalf of adults who have impaired hearing. These people, in many ways, are wishing to be recognized not simply as older persons, but as adults who have grown older, who have something to offer, and who do not want to be left alone. Their resolution to "not be a bother" and their resignation to "being old," in some cases, is the most logical choice in their minds for lack of alternatives. The audiologist can be a catalyst in developing a desire for self-enhancement.

The audiologist must be willing to work with these patients in a close professional manner and to accept the opportunity to assist in making a change in their lives. He or she must not be hesitant to intervene in a counseling role, but must recognize those instances when a patient's emotional problems are beyond the scope of the audiologist's service. For those persons, it is the responsibility of the audiologist to refer the individual to other appropriate counseling professionals.

Above all, the patient must be confident in the audiologist who is providing the hearing rehabilitation service. The patient must be aware that the audiologist or other service provider understands the communicative impact of presbycusis through his or her experience in working with other such patients. The patient must know that the audiologist feels that he or she can, indeed, be helped to communicate more efficiently through hearing rehabilitative services, and that feeling has justification on the basis of evaluation and potential benefit, not sympathy. A feeling of justified trust is the true key to motivational counseling.

Listen — talk — empathize — listen — encourage where appropriate — remember the status and age of the patient — provide support — counsel — listen — ask questions — expect answers — listen — provide guidance. Then, add an appropriate amount of *inspiration* for what may be the key to successful motivational counseling.

Adjusting/Manipulating the Listening Environment

As is noted in the "Process" section of this chapter, elderly patients initially are asked to establish priorities for situations in which they desire to function more efficiently. After this is completed, they are asked to choose one or two in which they most desire to learn to communicate more efficiently. They, of course, are requested to be reasonable in their selections. In this way, the hearing rehabilitation treatment program can be designed to meet their specific communication needs. In instances in which a patient's auditory difficulties are so severe that group sessions are not practical or cannot be tolerated by the patient, individual treatment is scheduled.

The goal, however, is to integrate the patient into a group situation as soon as possible, if at all possible. Another situation in which it is desirable that individual treatment be instituted is in the case of a patient whose priority communication environment is so unique as to warrant individual work.

A situation in point is a patient who was provided services individually by this author. His most difficult communication environment as a teacher in a middle school was his classroom. His treatment sessions, therefore, centered on physical/environmental adjustments in that specific room. The author worked with him individually on redesigning his classroom that was specific to his difficulties and strategies for communication in that environment. He had little difficulty in other more social environments.

Patient Discussions of Problem Environments

Problem-solving of difficult listening environments can be extremely productive. These sessions center on discussions of the patients' chosen prioritized communication environments. Priority environments most frequently center on church (understanding the minister or Sunday school teacher, or participating in church committee meetings), other environments in which groups of people meet socially, understanding what women or children are saying, or understanding what people are saying in environmentally distracting environments such as on the street corner, in a restaurant, or at the theater. The inevitable commonality of their choices allows for group sessions that are beneficial for everyone, as the majority of patients can enter into the discussions as they relate to them.

THE PROCESS

A problem specific to a certain environment, for example, is brought before the group by one of the therapy group members. The patient who presented the communication problem is asked to describe it in detail by giving examples of instances when it has occurred and the physical environment of each. As the physical environment is described, the therapist or the patient diagrams it on a chalkboard or flip chart as accurately as possible. The room or other physical environment is drawn, including windows, doors, partitions, furniture, and so on. The remainder of the group is then asked to give suggestions, as they see them, about how the patient could have adjusted to that communication environment by making physical adjustments, or making requests of the speaker, in their opinion, to resolve the patient's difficulty understanding what was being said.

As those suggestions are made, the therapist lists suggestions and illustrates the suggested adjustments on the previously drawn diagram; for example: (1) moving the patient's chair into a better situation for listening, (2) moving away from a bright window, (3) moving closer to a public address system speaker, (4) asking the person being conversed with to move closer, (5) walking out into a hallway where it is quieter, (6) asking the speaker to move closer to the microphone, or others.

Participation in this type of treatment activity can be extremely helpful and motivating. As the patient joins the group discussion by expanding on the explanation of the difficult environment and as questions or possible solutions are made, ways in which he or she may have been able to change that listening environment or future situations to his or her benefit become clearer. Others in the group also benefit because most may have found or may find themselves in a similar situation.

Creating Positive Assertiveness (Figure 5–2)

A trait that appears to become more typical as some people grow older is to become less assertive. This is particularly true of older adults who have been placed in a health care facility, or who have moved from their home to a retirement complex not of their own will, or who are trying to maintain their independence by remaining at home. Some may seem "stubborn," but those responses may be out of self-defense, perhaps because they

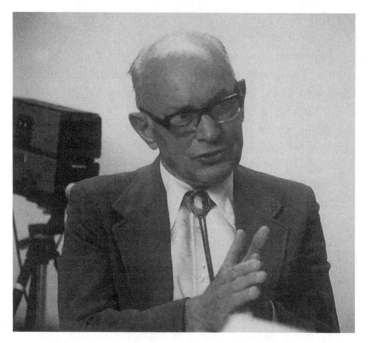

FIGURE 5–2. Assertiveness training brings out strengths patients may not realize they possess.

may not have heard or understood what was expected of them, or they may suspect that they are being "put-upon" rather than being allowed to make independent decisions about their life.

Furthermore, in all too many instances, older persons in health care facilities are not told what is going to be done to them, and find that things are being done *to* them rather than *for* them. Rather than continuing to react against the health care facility personnel and, thus, being listed as "uncooperative," they may become more passive.

Whether an older person is residing in a health care facility or in the community, it regrettably becomes more common for dramatic and sometimes unpleasant things to occur in that person's life. In light of the unexpected occurrences that may occur, it becomes easier to remain passive and wait rather than to become assertive and say "no," as they may be made to do it anyway. "Dad is getting stubborn in his old age," may be the label placed on the older person. Many older persons feel powerless because of a lack of independence. It is difficult to respond to a rapidly changing world when one does not possess the finances, transportation, physical mobility, quickness of analytical thought, or strength to manipulate one's environment.

Examples of Passive Behavior

One of this author's patients, a 78-year-old retired minister, was asked to chair a committee in his church because of his knowledge of religion. He was flattered to be asked to accept that position, but then shortly resigned because he could not understand what his committee members were saying. When I asked him why he did not ask the members to speak up, he said that he did once, but then they returned to their former way of speaking. When I asked him why he did not change the room arrangements so he could place himself in a more advantageous position for communication, he said that the room had been in that same arrangement for years, and he did not want to disrupt it. Those responses to potential change can defeat an otherwise potentially productive person.

Another example that illustrates the feelings of older adults who have impaired hearing is one that involved a 72-year-old female patient who had just returned from a lecture on Southeast Asia that she had been looking forward to attending for some time. She explained that the lecturer, a woman who had a rather soft voice, began talking to the audience through the public address system microphone, but then walked away from the microphone and stood beside the podium with the statement, "I'm sure that you can all hear me without the microphone."

The patient said that she hardly understood a word the speaker said throughout the next hour, but she was too embarrassed to leave the auditorium. When I asked her why she did not say, "Please use the microphone we are having difficulties hearing you," when the speaker moved away from the podium, her reply was that she just could not bring herself to do it. She wanted to, but was too embarrassed, "Besides," she said, "maybe I was the only person there who couldn't hear her."

When I asked her if she was important enough to warrant that speaker's consideration, this patient's response was simply, "I hope so." I said, "Don't you think that the microphone was placed there for a purpose? A public address system generally helps everyone to hear more comfortably. If you would have said something, I am sure that others in the audience would have been pleased that the presenter had returned to the podium and used the microphone." Her reply was that she had not thought of that. "But still," she said, "I didn't want to make a nuisance of myself. I'm just an old woman who can't hear very well." One of the audiologist's challenges is to work with the patient to change such attitudes of self-deprecation.

Learning to Help Themselves

The attitude just described is one that must be altered, if possible, if persons who posses impaired hearing are to learn to cope and function more efficiently in their communicative worlds. In light of the fact that some people are simply not willing to accommodate older adults who have impaired hearing or, perhaps are not aware of what accommodations can be made to facilitate communication, older persons must be taught ways to become assertive enough to make changes in their communication environments. Importantly, those include changes in the speaking habits of those with whom they desire to communicate.

Altering Passive Behaviors

As stated earlier, one way to alter passivity is by asking individual patients to describe difficult communication situations in which they have found themselves during the past week or month. The situation in which the 72-year-old woman found herself, as described above, is a prime example of the problems that are brought to the treatment sessions. Suggestions are brought forth by group members about similar experiences, and what they did to change them. When other group members courageously state what they would have done in that situation (e.g., to have told the woman speaker that, "I would appreciate it if you would use the microphone" in front of the audience), they are asked if they really would have done it? If they hold fast to their commitment, they are challenged to do it at the next lecture they attend when the speaker hesitates to use the microphone.

Occasionally, a group member returns after such an experience and triumphantly proclaims, "I did it!" On occasion, another member of the hearing rehabilitation treatment group who may have been in attendance at that meeting will confirm that the individual did a very nice job in changing a poor listening situation to a more pleasant one. Also, others at the meeting may have thanked our patient for asking the speaker to use the microphone by saying, "We just did not have the courage to speak up like that!" The triumph is great and does much toward encouraging the other group members to also become more assertive.

Other difficult situations brought before the groups may include family dinners, going to a noisy restaurant, talking to timid grandchildren, talking to one's attorney with other members of the family in attendance, and many others. The bywords in these treatment sessions are, "If those with whom we desire or must communicate do not seem to be accommodating, then we must assert ourselves by showing them *how* they can best communicate with us!" Suggestions or adjustments must be made without hesitation. To do otherwise is to "place ourselves back where we started." These are powerful and enjoyable treatment sessions that instill confidence in patients who may have not had confidence for some time.

Involvement of Family and Significant Others

The patient's family and significant others in the patient's life are critical elements for a successful hearing rehabilitation treatment program. This is particularly true if a patient's significant other is willing to become involved in the hearing rehabilitation process. This includes attending individual or group treatment sessions and participating in follow-up assignments.

A significant other's involvement in the hearing rehabilitation treatment process provides that person with a better understanding of the difficulties and frustrations with which the friend, spouse, or family member undergoing treatment is faced, particularly if he or she can attend the first sessions when discussions of hearing loss and difficult communication situations are emphasized. It further aids the patient's significant other to understand the commonality of communication difficulties when other patients discuss similar problems. The involvement prompts a realization that the communication difficulties that have arisen because of the auditory deficit are not only limited to their spouse, family member, or friend, but are found in others as well. One hopes that enhanced understanding can be passed on to others who are close to the patient.

This author frequently requests that those who attend the treatment sessions with individual patients be fit with ear plugs to at least experience to some degree what depressed hearing "sounds like." Some of the communicative frustrations revealed by the patients are often felt by the significant others at least during that brief period of time. It is explained to them, however, that ear plugs do not replicate the speech recognition problems being encountered by the person with whom they are attending the sessions, but simply demonstrate a mild to moderate loss of hearing acuity. Still, their use may enhance a feeling of empathy for the frustrations the hearing impaired person must feel.

One important byproduct of encouraging the involvement of a significant other in the hearing rehabilitation treatment program is that carryover of the treatment process into the everyday life of a patient can be greatly enhanced. If, for example, an older patient asserts him or herself before the remainder of the family by suggesting certain adjustments regarding seating arrangements for Thanksgiving dinner so that he or she can become involved in the conversation with greater efficiency, the significant other can reinforce and strengthen that positive step.

Furthermore, it is not as much fun to go to a restaurant or the movie alone. The significant other will not only strengthen and encourage carryover, but also make some potentially difficult situations more enjoyable. It helps to have someone there to back you up when the going gets rough!

One of the most discouraging aspects of the provision of any rehabilitative service to older patients is the lack of family involvement. In many instances, if a spouse has passed away, the remainder of the family may live quite a distance from the patient. Children may visit only once a year if the distance is great, and that may be for only a few days around a principal holiday, which can be a stressful time even for those with normal hearing. Even if grown children live in the same community, their desire for involvement with their parent on a social basis may be lacking, let alone a desire to become an important part of their mother's or father's rehabilitation program. The excuse generally is, "We just don't have time." In this remarkably advanced society, it is sad that we lose sight of the needs of our family. But, it seems to be the case, and alternatives for carryover support for older patients, in many cases, must be sought.

As stated earlier, a patient's spouse can be the most effective significant other, if the spouse is emotionally supportive of his or her husband or wife. If the spouse is not willing or capable of aiding in the support or carryover process, then a friend is appropriate and can be a most effective partner in the hearing rehabilitation process. In fact, at times it is common for people to discuss feelings with supportive friends prior to bringing them before a spouse or other family members. In any event, a close friend can be a very significant other.

A case to illustrate this point is that of a 70-year-old male patient who was provided hearing rehabilitation services by this author. He had been a widower for 4 years. On the first day of his group hearing rehabilitation program, he brought a female companion. Both loved to fish and were almost inseparable. Besides, as the old story bears out, she owned a boat and a camper from a previous relationship. They also both enjoyed attending social gatherings together, but the patient was experiencing great difficulty hearing and, in particular, understanding what was being said in those environments. His female companion was willing to explain what was being said, but was becoming frustrated at the consistency with which she had to function in the capacity of interpreter. In this instance, she attended all treatment sessions with the patient, she wearing her ear plugs and he his hearing aids. A great deal of warmth and understanding developed between them. As his ability to function communicatively increased, so did her willingness to assist in the treatment process through carryover. The assignments, which included experimentation at social gatherings, were carried out in an excellent manner. Problem situations that were to be discussed during treatment sessions lessened and, likewise, his dependence on his female companion for communicative support became less frequent. But, their relationship was enhanced.

The support and carryover by this significant other was instrumental in this patient's achievements in learning to use his residual hearing with greater efficiency, to use supplemental visual clues, and to change his difficult listening environments in constructive ways. Without such support and assistance, an audiologist may have greater difficulty facilitating such improvements.

ASSISTING OLDER ADULTS WHO POSSESS IMPAIRED HEARING

A hearing rehabilitation program for an older adult patient can include:

1. Assisting the older adult to become aware of the possible causes of hearing loss, and how it can impact on communication;

2. Ensuring that hearing enhancement through the acquisition of appropriate hearing aids or other listening systems;

3. Knowledge of the patient's desires and needs for communication;

4. Motivational counseling as an integral part of the process;

5. Learning how to manipulate or make positive change in one's *communicative environment* and the *speakers* in those environments to enhance communication;

6. Learning to become positively assertive;

7. Throughout everything listed, learning to use one's residual hearing and supplemental visual cues to enhance comprehension of verbal messages

To put this together into a meaningful hearing rehabilitation treatment program for an older adult is not really difficult. As a matter of fact, the process becomes quite logical once knowledge of the specific communicative needs of the patients have been confirmed.

The following is an example of an approach to hearing rehabilitation treatment for older adult patients, employing and intermingling the seven areas listed above. This process has been found effective for use with both confined and community-based older adults.

The Ongoing Hearing Rehabilitation Program: Reasons for Successful and Unsuccessful Treatment Programs

Some structure in the treatment process is desired by the majority of older patients. But, on the other hand, overly structured sessions can be counterproductive. For example, it is not uncommon for some audiologists to utilize traditional speechreading (lipreading) approaches that emphasize a progression from phoneme analysis to syllables, words, phrases, sentences, and stories. They generally begin to realize in a fairly short period of time that the patients who seemed motivated initially are attending "speechreading" sessions with less regularity. Soon they may cease attending altogether. Excuses can range from, "My family is coming to visit and I will be spending time with them," to "We have several church suppers coming up, and I have to help with them." It is embarrassing to see such persons downtown later with apparently nothing to do. Furthermore, they may call to tell your secretary that they really do not feel the need to come to "class" anymore, even though the audiologist knows that they have made little or no progress in treatment.

These patients are telling us something that we should receive loudly and clearly. That is, if they felt that hearing rehabilitation services were benefiting them, they probably would still be attending, as they evidently were motivated when they began.

A Must in Treatment

The hearing rehabilitation treatment programs *must* be geared to the specific needs of patients. If they are, they will take advantage of the services. However, if the audiologist begins the first session from a predetermined, prescriptive, approach, the patients will probably not remain interested in receiving the services. A few faithful patients might continue to attend, but they probably will leave the final session as able or unable to communicate with others they were in the beginning.

The therapist may wonder why these otherwise apparently alert older adults have not improved, even though they may say, "I enjoyed your 'class,'" and pat the audiologist on the shoulder. Furthermore, why would this audiologist have to coerce patients in health care facilities to attend hearing rehabilitation treatment sessions, or have to depend on a gracious activity director to bring them from their rooms to attend sessions that should be helping them cope in the everyday world more efficiently? It may be because the audiologist has lost sight of the fact that the treatment must be designed *with the needs of the patients in mind*. Other treatment procedures used by occupational therapists, physical therapists, speech-language pathologists, physicians and others are based on a treatment plan designed around the assessed *needs* of each patient. Why, then, are some audiologists still opening a "lipreading" lesson book and beginning at page 1 to provide services to patients who have varied and individual communication deficits and needs? Those speechreading books too often are used as "hymnals," and the session begins with the audiologist saying, "And for the next session we will turn to page 15." That is not treatment.

Individualizing the Approach

How does one develop a meaningful approach to hearing rehabilitation treatment for the older patient? More than 30 years ago Hardick (1977) described the basic characteristics of a successful hearing rehabilitation program for older adults. They are well defined and provide comprehensive guidance for those who intend to provide services for older patients, and in many ways are still current. Those characteristics are:

1. The program must be patient-centered.

2. The program must revolve around providing amplification and/or modifying a patient's communication environment.

3. All programs consist of individual therapy, with group sessions when appropriate.

4. The sessions should include normally hearing friends or relatives of the person who has impaired hearing so that strategies for improving their speech habits and/or the listening environments where communication usually takes place can be carried over into the life of the patient;

5. Hearing rehabilitation programs should be short term.

6. The program must be consumer-oriented.

7. Make use of "successful graduates" of the hearing rehabilitation program as resource people in therapy activities whenever possible.

These characteristics are extremely important for consideration prior to the initiation of hearing rehabilitation programs for older adults. They go far beyond the more traditional "lip-reading" procedures that continue to be employed by some. Even though some authors recommend group treatment for older patients, some will require individual services.

Other early patient-centered approaches to hearing rehabilitation are described by Alpiner, (1963); Alpiner and McCarthy (1987), Colton (1977), Colton and O'Neill (1976), Giolas (1994), Hull (1982, 1992, 1997, 2001, 2007), McCarthy and Alpiner (1978), M. Miller and Ort (1965), O'Neill and Oyer (1981), Sanders (1982, 1993), and others. The aspect stressed by these authors is that older adult patients possess needs that are specific to them, and each patient's hearing rehabilitation program must be centered on his or her needs and priorities.

If the ingredients presented on the previous pages are combined properly, a possible sequence of services emerges. An example of such a sequence is provided below.

Awareness of Reasons for Auditory Dysfunction

1. Understanding Hearing Loss

Facilitating an awareness of the reason for auditory communication difficulties through an understanding of the process of aging and its effect on the auditory mechanism is an important part of the hearing rehabilitation process. Included is a discussion of the central processing of auditory/speech/language information and the effect of aging on the speed and precision of that important function in communication particularly in noisy or otherwise distracting environments. The level of terminology is determined by the individual or group in question. The service provider is cautioned never to speak down to patients. It is important to use the correct technical terminology, but immediately explain it at the level of the persons involved. Clinicians must always remember that the patients are adults, no matter what their educational level or age. They deserve to be treated as such.

Charts need to be used in such discussions, perhaps along with pictures or PowerPoint presentations on the ear (Figure 5–3). If individuals in the group are severely hard of hearing, projected slides should be used only if enough light can remain in the room to facilitate the use of visual clues to observe the face and gestures of the service provider. Charts, diagrams, slides, and chalkboard drawings are used for these discussions, including presentations on: (1) the aging ear, (2) uses, benefits, and limitations of hearing aids, (3) environmental factors that affect communication, (4) poor speakers versus good speakers and what "good" and "poor" means, and (5) a general discussion of the aging process.

The basis for the first session or two is to facilitate a basis of understanding for the remainder of the treatment program, to develop a better understanding among the patients of what has occurred to them, and to assure them that in all probability they can improve, at least to some degree. Most persons leave

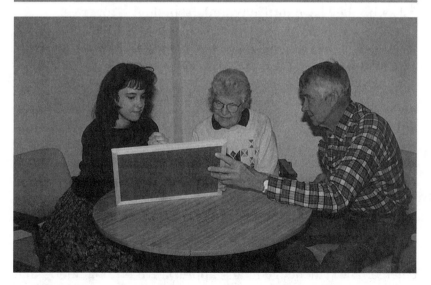

FIGURE 5–3. A spouse, family member, or significant other can reinforce an understanding of hearing loss and what it entails.

such session or sessions with a better understanding and greater acceptance of what is occurring to them and a desire to participate in the hearing rehabilitation treatment program.

It is key that a significant other in each patient's life should be encouraged to attend these sessions. Whether it be a spouse or a family member such as a child or a friend, he or she will gain much greater insight into the auditory/communication problems with which the person is attempting to cope.

2. Prioritized Communicative Needs

The second step in the hearing rehabilitation treatment programs is, as stated earlier, to ask each patient to list those difficulties in communication that most affect him or her. The Wichita State University Communication Appraisal and Priorities Profile (CAPP), as presented in Figure 5–4, can be used in this process. They may include specific communication environments such as a meeting room, church, certain restaurant, table arrangement at their child's home, and so on. They also may list certain individuals who they have difficulty understanding.

The next step is for patients to prioritize those situations or persons, from most important to least important, and, if they had their choice, in which of those would they most like to improve first. They are asked, of course, to be realistic in their final choices. For some, the choice is an obvious one. For others, it may be more difficult. It is important to note, however, that if gains are made in one category, there is a good probability that patients will observe improvement in other related circumstances.

They are asked to discuss their choices, present a situation in which they had difficulty, and explain what prompted them to make those choices. Particularly in a group situation, it is interesting to note the general consistency of priority areas that emerge. The patients generally appreciate the camaraderie that develops out of these discussions. For the first time, many of them realize that they are not the only ones who have difficulty in these environments.

The WSU Communication
Appraisal and Priorities Profile

Date_____

Name_____ Age_____ Sex____

Address_____ Phone_____

Please indicate below those situations in which you are able to communicate best, those that are difficult for you in some instances, and those that are a definite problem. Under "explain," please tell us more if you desire, such as certain instances when you experience more difficulty than others, certain types of speakers, certain places, and so on.

	No problems	Only in specific instances	Definite problem	Priority
1. At parties or other social events	____	____	____	____
Explain_____				
_____				
2. At the dinner table	____	____	____	____
Explain_____				
_____				
3. On the telephone	____	____	____	____
Explain_____				
_____				
4. At home	____	____	____	____
Explain_____				
_____				
5. With males	____	____	____	____
Explain_____				
_____				
6. With females	____	____	____	____
Explain_____				
_____				

FIGURE 5–4. The WSU Communication Appraisal and Priorities Profile (CAPP).

3. Poor Speakers and Poor Listening Environments

This author tells his patients that we all live in a world of poor speakers and places that are not meant for communication. We do, indeed! Therefore, patients rightfully can put part of the blame for their auditory/communicative difficulties on others who display poor speech habits, or the places with poor acoustics where they go to worship, attend the theater, or visit family. Those are acknowledged and discussed. The discussion centers on the fact that there indeed are many poor speakers in this world. A demonstration of some of the habits that interfere with efficient communication is appropriate. Patients generally immediately recognize poor speaking habits. Even though there are many poor speakers, persons with impaired hearing must develop ways to cope in those communication environments. The encouraging acknowledgment that they can, in many instances, manipulate such difficult situations in order to function more efficiently in them, and that they will be working on those situations, ends the discussion on a positive note.

These generally do not consume more than 1 or 2 full-hour sessions, although the first part of each session consists of airing of difficult listening situations that they found themselves in during the previous week. Those are discussed and resolved to the degree possible. The discussions of priority difficulties and circumstances that interfere with efficient communication should not be curtailed, however, because the airing of frustrations and concerns will greatly facilitate future progress. For many, this may be the first time those concerns have been discussed. To prematurely conclude such discussions simply on the basis of a rigid schedule can stifle the airing of emotions and adjustment that may have otherwise been made.

4. On Becoming Assertive

Weekly assignments for each patient are made and include noting a communication situation in which they had particular difficulty that, in the end, interfered with communication. Patients are to bring the specifics of the situation to the next treatment session for presentation and discussion. They are asked to write down descriptions of situations, and diagram the physical environment if necessary (or simply recall them as accurately as possible). Each patient (or in the case of individual treatment, the patient) presents the difficult situation they experienced, if one has been noted. It is imperative that the patient who was involved in the situation be the one who presents it and not the significant other who may accompany the patient.

After a thorough presentation, with diagrams drawn on a black or white board, the situation is discussed by the group (or in the event of individual treatment, by the patient, the audiologist, and the accompanying significant other, if he or she was involved). Suggestions regarding possible ways the patient might have manipulated the communication environment to his or her best advantage, including the physical environment or the speaker, are made by the group under the guidance of the service provider and are accepted as viable or discarded.

As stated by this author previously (Hull, 2007, 2011), insights into ways of manipulating the communication environment to their best advantage, along with methods of coping with and adjusting to frustrating listening environments, in turn, are developed among patients under the guidance of the audiologist. This form of self- and group analysis is an extremely important part of the hearing rehabilitation program. Patients, then, are helped to develop their own insights into methods of adjusting to situations where communication is difficult. If, for some reason, they find that it is impossible for them to make the necessary adjustments, perhaps they can, in a positive-supportive-assertive manner, decrease their difficulty by requesting that others make certain adjustments in the listening environment or manner of speaking. Perhaps, they could request that the physical environment be adjusted so that they can function more efficiently in it, or they can "take charge" and make adjustments on their own.

It becomes difficult for some older patients to develop even mildly assertive behaviors. They do not want to be noticed as a "demanding" older person. Many do feel rather vulnerable, perhaps feeling that the people who invited them to a party did so more out of obligation than desire. They may feel that if they request that those who are seeking to converse with them move to a quieter place to talk, or request that someone change the position of his or her chair to be in a better position to talk then, perhaps, the hosts will feel that it is more trouble than it is worth to invite them again. In light of such fears, it can become logical to avoid that possibility by simply remaining quiet and being fearful that if asked a question, he or she might be embarrassed by answering inappropriately. Those fears are occasionally brought forth by patients and should be discussed as they arise.

Examples of those discussions include one that was initiated by one of this author's patients who was being seen on a group basis. The woman in question was discussing a situation involving another woman with whom she had morning coffee on an almost daily basis for a number of years. The patient's complaint was that her friend was an incessant gum chewer and, as the chewing continued as she talked, it interfered with precise articulation, and her ability to understand what she was saying. Her friend interpreted the patient's inability to understand what she was saying to be the result of her impaired hearing, not her imprecise manner of speaking resulting from her enthusiastic gum chewing, which was compounded by the patient's hearing loss. This apparent misinterpretation of the situation infuriated my patient. But, she continued the morning coffee time, because there were few other women her age in that geographic area and, besides, they had been friends since childhood.

This woman's major concern was how to tell her friend that her manner of speaking and gum chewing had, for several years, interfered with her ability to understand what she was saying and, in the end, made what might have been a pleasant conversation, a difficult one. She was particularly afraid to say anything because of the embarrassment her friend might feel because the situation had been going on for so long and nothing had previously been said. "Almost like," as the patient said, "being associated with a person for a long time and never knowing her name.

As time passes, you become increasingly embarrassed about asking her name, particularly when she knows yours." The suggestions that came from the group varied from an enthusiastic, "Tell her that if she wants to talk to you, to take her gum out of her mouth!" to a timid, "If you value your friendship, maybe it is best to say nothing and simply tolerate the situation." The latter suggestion was discarded. The ultimate conclusion simply was to tell the truth.

It was the consensus of the group that they would respect their own friend more if he or she would say something like, "You know, we've been friends for a long time. You realize, as I do, that I have some difficulty hearing what people say to me. I have particular difficulty with men who wear mustaches or beards, people who do not move their lips enough, or people who talk with their hand near their mouth, as I depend on seeing the face of persons with whom I am talking. You know, I have difficulty understanding what you say sometimes and I think that I may have discovered why. I know that you like to chew gum a great deal and, like me, it helps my mouth not to become so dry. I do think, however, that because you, probably not realizing it, chew your gum while we are talking, it doesn't allow me to see your lips move properly and, besides, you aren't able to talk as plainly when you chew it so hard. I just bet that if you don't chew gum while we are having our coffee, I will be able to understand you better and we'll have a nicer time talking. Do you want to give it a try?" *Positive assertiveness* are the two key words in this instance. For that patient, the strategy she and the remainder of the group determined as most effective did prove to be successful and she maintained the friendship.

5. Other Topics to Facilitate Communication (Table 5–1)

Other topics for discussion and for the development of communicative strategies may include: (1) weekly socials at private homes where the furniture arrangements interfere with efficient communication. Some, as experienced through this author's work with older patients, involve: (2) the table arrangement at

TABLE 5–1. Topics For Discussion Stressed During Treatment Sessions

- Relaxation under stressful conditions.

- Confidence that clients can piece together the thought of the verbal message, even though not all of it was heard.

- Remembering that because of their normal language function and their knowledge of the predictability of American English, they can determine what is being said if supplemental visual cues are used along with as much auditory information as is possible under the environmental circumstance.

- Knowledge that other people in the same environment also may be having difficulty understanding what others are saying and that they also may or may not be coping successfully with the stress.

- Freedom to manipulate the communication environment as much as possible by, for example, asking the person with whom they are speaking to move with them to a slightly quieter corner where they can talk with greater ease or move his or her chair to a more advantageous position so the speaker can be seen and/or heard more clearly, or other positive steps to enhance communication.

- Remembering that if difficulty in a communication environment seems to be increasing, and feelings of concern or nervousness begin to become evident, they should feel free to interrupt the conversation and talk about the noise or the activity around them that seems to be causing the difficulties. The other person will probably agree with that observation and, in talking about it, feelings of stress may be reduced and communication may be enhanced.

one patient's son's home where they usually had Thanksgiving dinner, (3) the television set at a male patient's friend's home, (4) the seating arrangement and acoustics at a church meeting room, and others. Even though the discussions and thought-provoking suggestions generally provide guidance to the individual whose situation is being discussed, they also provide insights for the remainder of the group on how they, too, may be able to manipulate similar communicative environments.

These assertiveness sessions can be extremely stimulating for the patients and for their significant other who may be in attendance. Patients have told this author that those sessions are probably the most valuable for them, particularly because we are working and sharing on behalf of their problems in communication. As patients identify with other patients' difficult communication situations and relate to solutions as they see them, insights into solutions for their own difficult situations emerge and are strengthened.

Self-confidence reawakens when patients return to state that the solution developed during the previous session did not work as planned, but with a few adjustments developed by him or herself, it did! Most older patients, no matter the level of hearing impairment or how distraught they may be as a result of their difficulties in hearing, can benefit from these assertiveness sessions. The topics of "self-worth" and, "I'm important too" that become a part of the discussions are an extremely important part of the total hearing rehabilitation program.

Environmental Design

Hull (2001 and 2011) has described avenues for educating older patients who have hearing impairment regarding techniques and strategies of environmental design. This involves modifying the acoustical/environmental design of their homes, offices, and other communicative environments to their listening/communicative advantage. Training also involves how to make modifications in those and other situations in which they find themselves, including social environments, meetings, and business environments that otherwise may have placed them at a communicative disadvantage. These can be very powerful hearing rehabilitation sessions that provide patients with tangible methods for modifying their most difficult communication situations.

Speaking to Older Adults

The following are "Ten Commandments" for speaking to older adults who possess impaired hearing. They, of course, are not set in stone, because every older adult with impaired hearing is different. They are, however, general principles that can be kept in mind when talking to them.

1. Speak to the person at a distance no greater than 6 feet, and no closer than 2 feet;

2. Use light to its utmost, but focus the light on the face of the speaker, *not* the listener;

3. Speak at the visual level of the listener. If the older adult is using a wheelchair, for example, the speaker should sit or kneel so that her or his face is visible;

4. No matter how much hearing impairment the older adult possesses, *do not* speak directly into their ear. This not only tends to distort the sounds of speech, but the intensity distorts the listener's auditory system;

5. Speak at a natural rate. Do not slow speech to an unnatural rate. As most adults speak too rapidly for the older central auditory system to process accurately, simply slow the rate of speech slightly. This author has timed news broadcasters, for example, at speaking rates of up to 200 words per minute (wpm), and typical adults speaking regularly at rates of 170 to 180 wpm. The older adults' central auditory system can process speech accurately when it is spoken at a rate of *between 120 and 130 wpm*. Speakers including family members, pastors of churches, news broadcasters, and all others should practice speaking at no greater than 130 wpm so that all persons, older and younger, will understand what they are saying with greater efficiency.

6. Speak at a slightly louder than average intensity, but not so loud that it distorts your manner of speaking;

7. Do not speak to the back of the listener. If you are approaching the older adult, walk around so that you are visible and make sure that you have the listener's attention before beginning to speak;

8. Speak in short sentences. If what you are saying involves directions or instructions, break them into short concise statements and wait until you are sure the person understands before moving on to the next statement;

9. If the older adult seems confused by your statement and answers inappropriately, do not ignore the confusion by simply moving on to the next. If one statement is not understood, use other words to describe what you were saying. *Do not* use the same words over and over again.

10. Above all, remember that you are speaking to an adult.

SUMMARY

It is important for older patients to be given the opportunity to make decisions regarding areas of communication in which they desire to improve. Even though many may feel discouraged because of the embarrassing difficulties they experience in their attempts at understanding what others are saying, they have communicative priorities that must be addressed through their hearing rehabilitation programs.

As adults who probably possessed normal hearing during the majority of their lives and whose case histories may reveal nothing more than that they have become older, they deserve to participate in the decisions regarding their treatment program. However, guidance must be provided by the audiologist.

CHAPTER 6

Older Adults in Health Care Facilities

INTRODUCTION

Approximately 7% of all persons beyond age 65 years reside in health care facilities (Ignatavicius & Bayne, 1995). Of the some 40 million persons over age 65 years, that percentage represents more than 2.8 million persons (Health Care Financing Administration, 2004). Placement rates for the young-old persons aged 65 to 74 seem to have fallen recently, especially for older men, many of whom are re-marrying. But, among persons aged 75 to 84, rates have increased, particularly for women. Older women who are most likely to be placed in a health care facility are poor, or widowed-living alone, and very old. Earlier, in 1972, Atchley reported that over 14% of persons age 85 or over were living in various levels of healthcare facilities. Of those, most were placed in nursing homes or other personal care facilities. On the other hand, in 1987, Stone, Cafferata, and Sangl reported that 21% of persons age 85 years and beyond were recipients of specialized care either in nursing homes, by home health care agencies, or by family. In 1996, the Administration on Aging placed the number of persons over age 70 years who were residing in nursing homes at more than 2 million. Currently, these numbers have, as persons continue to live to greater ages, reached over 2.5 million.

In 1996, more than 20% of older persons were limited in their activity because of chronic health conditions, that is, 14% for persons age 65 to 74 years, 26% for persons 75 to 84 years, and 48% for those beyond age 85 years (Administration on Aging, 2002). Furthermore, about 92% of older persons wear glasses and approximately 60% have hearing impairment to a sufficient degree to interfere with their activities of daily living (Administration on Aging, 2002; Hull, 2009). According to Hull (2001), approximately 92% of persons residing in health care facilities possess hearing impairment of sufficient degree to interfere with their activities of daily living. In an earlier survey, Schow and Nerbonne (1980) found the incidence of hearing loss among health care facility residents to be 80%.

Although many of these persons will, for all practical purposes, remain confined for the remainder of their lives because of chronic illness and other physical or mental problems, many can benefit from hearing rehabilitation services from an audiologist. They deserve the opportunity for enhanced communicative skills in spite of impaired hearing and to experience the heightened social and personal communication that may result. Furthermore, with effective in-service education for health care facility personnel on the topics of hearing impairment, the use of hearing aids, and communication with older adults who have hearing impairment, the daily lives of elderly persons, and the staff, within a health care facility can be enhanced. One hopes these services will be coordinated with educational programming for elderly persons and their families.

HEALTH CARE FACILITIES

Before this discussion of services for confined older people proceeds, a description of what is meant by "health care facility" is appropriate.

Health care facility is a currently accepted term denoting any facility that provides long- or short-term residential care for older adults who require medical or other health services other than that provided by hospitals. The facilities may provide intensive care services, including 24-hour-a-day nursing care for posthospitalized stroke patients, or simply a place to live near nursing or other health care.

Outpatient Residential Facilities

These facilities may include apartment or condominium living for ambulatory older adults. The apartments, or condominiums, in this instance, are a part of a health care facility, perhaps in a separate wing or simply on the same grounds. Immediate health care is usually a button-push away. Older persons who reside in an outpatient or residential facility may have been ill enough at some recent time to desire the proximity of those services. Some of these facilities most nearly resemble what are generally called "retirement communities." The only difference is they are generally a part of a larger health care facility complex representing various levels of care.

Short-Term Care Facilities

Many health care facilities have an intensive care or a skilled nursing wing or may be an intensive-care or skilled nursing facility. These generally are considered short-term care facilities. A stroke patient, for example, when known to be recovering, but is still too ill to return to his or her own home because of the need for rather constant monitoring and nursing care, may be released from the hospital and taken to the short-term care facility. The stay may be only a few days or may last for several weeks where services such as occupational therapy, physical therapy, speech therapy will be provided. These facilities play an important role, not only for recuperative purposes, but also as an alterative to higher cost extended hospital stays. For stroke patients and others who may require other services, rehabilitation personnel such as occupational therapists, audiologists, speech-language pathologists, and others are generally available, at least on a contractual basis.

When placed in a short-term facility, it is expected that the patient will be released within a fairly short time. The most desirable destination is the patient's home. Unfortunately, however, for some older adults, the destination is to an intermediate or long-term care facility, for lack of other alternatives.

Intermediate and Long-Term Care Facilities

The most frequently observed facilities for older adults are often called "nursing homes." They are facilities where older adults reside who may require nursing or other health care. The primary reason for placement is generally a health or other debilitating problem. However, intermediate care facilities all too frequently become long term in nature. For example, placement in these health care facilities may be because: (1) no place else to live, (2) a spouse has passed away and the elderly survivor fears living alone, or (3) most frustrating to older persons, the elderly person's family "feels that it is best." As one older woman told this author, "I thought my daughter was out looking for an apartment for me and I ended up here!"

These facilities offer a room (often with a roommate), balanced meals, some social and recreational activities, and a nursing staff. Larger health care facilities may have a social services director, an activity director, and rehabilitative services such as occupational therapy, speech-language therapy, and physical therapy. Some facilities are Medicare and/or Medicaid-approved, but for those programs to provide payment for services and residence, a medically related problem must be the reason for placement in the facility. Furthermore, some health care facilities do not want to be approved by either program because of the relatively low rate of reimbursement for care of the residents, particularly from Medicaid.

THE RESIDENTS OF HEALTH CARE FACILITIES

The older adults who are placed in skilled or intensive-care wings of health care facilities or in skilled nursing care facilities are there because of specific health or mental reasons. They may have been transferred from a hospital to the skilled nursing facility because they are still too weak or unable to care for themselves at home, but well enough to be released from the hospital. It is anticipated that the facility and the 24-hour-per-day nursing care that is available, in that respect, will be the "halfway house" for the patient between hospitalization and home. In some instances, however, because of lack of sufficient recovery, some older patients must be transferred to an extended-care facility because they are not able to care for themselves sufficiently to live at home and, furthermore, there may not be others at home to help the person. Therefore, the adult is placed in a longer term health care facility so that the necessary services for daily needs are available. In all too many instances, an elderly person views such placement as terminal. The latter represents a fear that can interfere with the person's desire for rehabilitative services if those are needed. The audiologist and other health care professionals must be aware of this, as well as other responses and feelings that can interfere with patient desire for supportive services.

Reasons for Placement

What are the reasons for placement in extended care facilities? Because placement for any reason can result in a lessening of desire for self-maintenance and/or improvement, the audiologist or other provider of services should be aware of them. According to early discussions by Atchley (1972), and Gatz, Bengston, and Blum (1990), the major factor in placement of persons in health care facilities (nursing homes or other residences) appears to be their state of mental or physical health, their previous residential setting, or the family system. Older people in nursing and other health care facilities tend not to have a spouse or children who live nearby, although many have living children. Indications are that many older people would be able to avoid institutionalization if they had relatives to help care for them (Gatz et al., 1990), and if they had adequate finances. A breakdown in the support system appears to be the primary cause for placement in nursing homes or other forms of residential facilities. Others include loss of residence because of urban renewal projects, or perhaps a child who has urged them to sell a house (that according to the child is just too much for the elderly family member to care for).

The placement of an older adult in a health care facility does not generally occur rapidly. A series of events usually take place prior to placement. Among those events are serious illness or a serious fall. The events may include attempts at placing the person with relatives who, in the end, find the older person to be too much of an emotional or financial burden. For whatever reason, placement in a health care facility (nursing home) was felt to be a necessity and the factors leading to that decision frequently may affect the morale of both the older person and his or her family.

The Impact of Placement

As the majority of older adults view residence in a nursing home as a last resort—in all probability terminal placement—its impact on an older person can have a number of negative implications that the audiologist or other health professionals who may attempt to provide diagnostic and rehabilitative services must recognize. The negative effects include:

1. Depression.

2. Loneliness.

3. A growing lack of desire to receive rehabilitative services when they may be indicated.

4. The shock and stress associated with the move to a nursing home from a residence where the person may have lived for many years.

5. A lessening of self-image or self-realization due to the routine of the nursing home.

6. Gradual dependency on persons who, no matter how caring and helpful, are strangers.

7. A lessening of awareness of occurrences in the outside world due to the isolating effect of the nursing home.

8. Personality changes resulting from isolation and/or certain medications.

9. A loss of independence.

10. A loss of personal control including who his or her roommate will be, time for sleeping and eating, and other aspects of life.

11. The depressing influence of illness.

12. The dehumanization of people which can occur in more institutionalized nursing homes.

13. A lack of personal stimulation, which occurs from a loss of close interpersonal communication.

14. A reduction of sensory capabilities that comes with age, including sense of smell, touch, sight, and hearing.

SUMMARY

These effects and many others not mentioned are difficult to overcome. As a result, the elderly resident of a nursing home may not readily accept an audiologist's or any service provider's services. It requires a service provider and family who will work with the confined older adult in positive and constructive ways to instill in the older adult a desire for rehabilitation services. Chapter 7 provides information on procedures for serving older adults with impaired hearing who reside in various levels of health care facilities.

CHAPTER 7

Serving the Special Needs of Older Adults with Impaired Hearing in Health Care Facilities

INTRODUCTION

The large population of persons who have hearing impairment who reside in various levels of health care facilities were, for many years, either ignored or avoided because it was felt they possessed little rehabilitative potential. Others believed they were experiencing so many other problems that it was probably best to leave them alone.

In the past, and in some instances still currently, many hearing assessment and rehabilitation services on behalf of elderly nursing home patients have been provided as parts of practicum experiences by graduate students in audiology training programs. In the great majority of instances, however, the students did not possess the insights into aging and aging persons needed to provide effective services. Rather, they may have begun with "Lesson Number One" in a book of speechreading lessons and proceeded to provide "speechreading instruction" that may have had little or no meaning for the patients involved. The majority of patients, then, had to be "rounded-up" before each weekly session, and the gradually disillusioned graduate student clinician wondered why so many would not leave their room to come to "class." The student clinician may have felt that the book of speechreading lessons must contain *something* that would benefit the older patients or else it would not have been written. More importantly, the patients were told that the hearing rehabilitation program might help them learn to communicate more efficiently with others in spite of their impaired hearing, only to realize later that it did not. It is no wonder, then, that audiologists graduating from training programs may have had little desire to initiate audiology service programs in health care facilities. The fact is that many of those graduate students did not have had a positive practicum experience in that setting, and found it to be less than stimulating. The residents probably felt the same way!

Addressing the Needs of Health Care Facility Residents

It is important to remember that residents of health care facilities are individuals who have specific goals and needs. Among the 92% of health care facility residents who possess some degree of hearing impairment, the sense of need and urgency for interpersonal communication is as great as for anyone else. After all, verbal communication is one of the traits that identifies us as human. The isolation that occurs as the result of impaired hearing can be even more devastating to persons who are already isolated because of their confinement in a nursing home. Their sense of urgency to break through the barriers to communication caused by an inability to hear and understand what others are saying or, at least, to watch television or the HFC Saturday evening movie and understand what is being said may be much greater than exhibited by their statements or emotions. They, further, may have suppressed a desire to accept services that may benefit them since they may feel that perhaps nothing will help at their late stage of life.

However, if the hearing rehabilitation services are geared toward the specific priorities of the patient, the probability that the procedures will benefit the residents of health care facilities will be greater. Before beginning rehabilitation, however, the patients must be encouraged to develop a desire to at least "give it a try." Within reason, depending on their state of health and mental competence, improvements can be made if they also accept the opportunity to participate.

Above and beyond the service aspect is the important fact that the audiologist is working with adults, no matter what their age or temperament. They are adults who, beyond their desire or control, have become older. And with age, an increasing inability to efficiently hear and understand what others are saying has added to the isolation and depression they may be experiencing. If the audiologist offers the time, energy, and commitment to learn about the process of aging and listen to what his or her patients are saying about their needs, desires, and concerns, then viable aural rehabilitation treatment programs can be developed.

Developing Realistic Expectations

Another important aspect of this fascinating work must be acknowledged. That is, audiologists who provide the hearing services must be realistic in their efforts and expectations when serving this population. No matter how much we would like to effectively serve all persons, there ar some who do not have the potential to benefit from hearing rehabilitation services, whereas others may benefit only marginally. On the other hand, the audiologist must refrain from providing services only on behalf of those who will benefit most to the exclusion of those who may benefit slightly. Even a terminally ill, bedridden person's last weeks or months may be brightened by a health care facility nursing staff that has learned from the audiologists' in-services how to communicate more efficiently with persons who have impaired hearing, and an assistive listening device may enhance their ability to hear or talk with their family. This, in itself, can be a significant service. These are *quality*, not quantity, of life issues.

DETERMINING THE NEED FOR SERVICES

Establishing the Benefits

In most health care facilities, it can be assumed that at least a sizable number of persons who reside there possess impaired hearing and can benefit from some aspect of an assessment and hearing rehabilitation program. The benefits of initiating an aural rehabilitation program should be presented to the director and his or her staff. The benefits that can be stressed in that meeting include:

1. The fact that effective in-service education can enhance communication between health care facility personnel and residents who have impaired hearing and, thus, ease one reason for frayed nerves on both parts.

2. Recommendations for alterations in the furniture arrangement in a lounge area or other central gathering place that can enhance communication. This, alone, can be of great service to a health care facility. Otherwise, residents may avoid an important area where the greatest amount of activity and communication was supposed to take place.

3. Effective hearing aid counseling and orientation programs can provide the impetus for previously inefficient users of hearing aids to benefit from them in their daily activities.

4. An effective assessment program can identify persons who have hearing impairment who may have been thought to be noncommunicative or "confused" for other reasons.

5. For some, a well-designed hearing rehabilitation treatment program can provide enhanced communicative skill, which can reduce stress for both for caregivers and the patient. For others, the hearing rehabilitation program may consist of discussions of patients' most difficult communication environments and suggestions for changing the physical environment, or instructing the persons with whom they have difficulty communicating on how to speak with greater clarity.

These programs, if geared toward patients' specific communication needs, can be extremely beneficial for confined elderly residents. It is also generally found that most persons in the health care facility environment can benefit from at least some aspect of these services either directly or indirectly.

Surveying for Hearing Impairment

The determination of the need for any of the services discussed previously must begin with a survey of the residents of the health care facility and, in specific terms, a presentation of the results of the survey to the health care facility administration. These include the director, the head of nursing, the activity director, and the social services director. It is suggested that all residents who can respond to a hearing evaluation be included in the hearing testing.

A typical hearing screening at a fixed intensity level has generally not been found to be a satisfactory method for use in a health care facility because such large numbers fail. An efficient procedure includes establishing pure-tone thresholds and the use of impedance audiometry to confirm the type of loss. Even if a quiet environment for assessment can be found, the use of impedance audiometry is important because even low noise levels can interfere with bone-conduction hearing assessments.

For those who are found to have impaired hearing, assessment of speech recognition ability with and without visual clues provides relevant information for initial discussions with the health care facility staff about each individual patient's disability and the need for aural rehabilitation services. Speech recognition, in the absence of a sound-treated room and audiometer with speech capabilities, can be assessed with relative accuracy by live voice, with the audiologist seated approximately 4 to 6 feet from the patient. Monosyllabic words, CID Everyday Sentences, and a brief conversation with and without visual clues administered at a comfortable listening level for the patient, can provide some important information about the person's speech recognition abilities. However, this should only be conducted by a skilled audiologist who can interpret the results of those rather informal testing procedures.

Presentation of Survey Results

Results of the survey are presented to the administration of the health care facility and, if that facility is a part of a corporate body, a representative of the corporation. If the administration is convinced that a hearing rehabilitation program is warranted and desired, then the program format is outlined.

The survey, alone, will provide important information for the health care facility staff. Residents who previously may have been described as confused and/or disoriented may be found to possess a severe enough hearing impairment to account for at least a portion of that behavior. Modifications in patterns of communication by health care facility staff alone may result in positive behavior change on the part of both the staff and those residents. Those modifications in communication strategies by the staff, for example, can result from instruction through a staff in-service program. An elderly man, previously described as stubborn, inattentive, withdrawn, and antisocial, may begin to interact in a more positive and interactive manner when communication with staff is likewise enhanced. Others may demonstrate positive personality change as the result of properly fitted hearing aids, combined with modifications of speaking habits by health care facility staff as the result of an effective in-service program. Being able to hear one's TV by way of an assistive listening device so that the resident can once again enjoy her or his favorite shows can be a positive life changing event.

With information on the incidence, severity, and communicative impact of hearing loss within the health care facility to be presented to the administration, a full assessment and aural rehabilitation program can be outlined and initiated. This includes a discussion of the possible positive impact of a viable hearing rehabilitation program on the residents, on the health care facility staff, and on the other programs within the facility.

Patient Records

Records of progress for each patient must be maintained on an ongoing basis, along with records of physician, staff, family contact, and referrals. Records of social progress, continuing service, medical records, staff notification of audiometric test results, physician and family notification, and progress in the aural rehabilitation program are integral parts of the audiologist's record-keeping procedures. Such reports should be kept both in the patient's master file in the health care facility and as a part of the audiologist's file on each patient.

Patient Care Plan

A patient care plan is developed in cooperation with the audiologist, the speech-language pathologist, social services personnel, and other staff who have daily contact with the person, including the activities director. The plan contains the goals and objectives for each aural rehabilitation patient, along with methods and approaches and the problem or concern. An example of a patient care plan is found in Figure 7–1.

KENTON MANOR

AUDIOLOGY CARE PLAN

RESIDENT: ROOM LOCATION:

A. PROBLEM OR CONCERN:

B. GOALS OF CARE TEAM:

C. METHODS AND APPROACHES:

D. COMMENTS:

NAME:

TITLE:

DATE:

FIGURE 7–1. Example of patient care plan for aural rehabilitation programs in a health care facility.

Continuing Service Records

Continuing service records must be maintained on an ongoing basis. Each note, dated and signed, relates, for example, to progress in specific aural rehabilitation efforts, a contact made by the audiologist with that patient for hearing aid maintenance, statements regarding communicative progress, or a contact by a family member or the patient's physician.

Communication Progress Forms

Communication progress forms are also integral to the record-keeping efforts on behalf of the health care facility program. The patient's baseline of communicative behavior is noted on each form. Each form for each member of the evaluation team is placed in a patient's file. As each person notes specific changes in communicative behavior, they are noted on his or her own form for each patient. At weekly or monthly staff meetings, the ratings for each patient are compared, and a consensus as to progress or lack of it is noted in the patient's continuing service record.

Reimbursement for Services

In discussing the auditory assessment program, the aural rehabilitation program, and reimbursement issues with the health care facility administration, it should be emphasized that Medicare and, in some states, Medicaid cover auditory diagnostic evaluations, including special assessment procedures, in accordance with billing procedures and charges that are reasonable and typical in that geographic area. The testing must be justified on an individual basis. Routine testing may not be reimbursed. Audiologists who are certified, or are eligible for certification as audiologists by the American Speech-Language-Hearing Association, or licensed by states having licensure laws, are eligible to become Medicare approved providers of audiology services by award of a Medicare provider number. If the health care facility is Medicare-approved, its own accounting office can bill for the service. In whatever manner, an agreement for the method of reimbursement for services should, in all instances, be arranged before the initial survey.

THE ONGOING HEARING REHABILITATION PROGRAM

In-Service Training of Health Care Facility Personnel and Families of the Residents

In-service training for health care facility administration, staff, and the residents' families not only supports an assessment and aural rehabilitation treatment program, but also provides carryover of the treatment aspects into the daily life of the residents. In-service provides administration, staff, and families with insights into: (1) the cause and effects of presbycusis on residents' ability for communication, (2) the resulting psychosocial impact, (3) the structure of the aural rehabilitation program, (4) what hearing aids can and cannot do, (5) troubleshooting procedures for hearing aid malfunction, and (6) methods for more efficient communication with residents who have hearing impairment.

Included during staff/administration in-services are discussions of individual residents who are involved as patients in the program. Discussions include: (1) the hearing impairment those patients possess; (2) the potential impact of the hearing impairment on their communicative function; (3) their progress (or lack of it) as a result of the hearing rehabilitation treatment program; and (4) the development of plans for follow-through and carryover of those patients' programs into their daily lives in the health care facility. The health care facility staff, including the director of nurses, activity director, physical therapist, occupational therapist, and other personnel, including the cooks and custodians, can all be vital forces in the carryover process. This, importantly, includes the families of the residents if they are available to attend.

Techniques offered through in-service for more efficient communication with older persons who have hearing impairment can enhance the lives of the staff, the residents' families, and the residents. It is generally found, to everyone's relief, that some of the emotional encounters resulting from futile attempts at communication between residents who have hearing impairment and staff members are sometimes soothed after utilization of the techniques for communication that the staff learned during in-service and that the elderly patients are learning during their treatment sessions.

Topics That In-Service Training Should Include

1. The basic structure of the auditory mechanism and possible reasons as to the causes of presbycusis.

2. The manifestations of presbycusis and its potential impact on an elderly person's ability to function communicatively. This discussion includes presentations of audiometric configurations and examples of what the patient who possesses presbycusis might hear, compared with hearing that is normal.

3. Hearing aids, their uses and misuses, are discussed relative to what hearing aids are, what they sound like, what they can do, and what they cannot do. The reasons why some persons cannot benefit from hearing aids are also discussed, along with the necessity for a thorough hearing aid evaluation by a licensed audiologist.

4. Instruction on the use of hearing aids, placing the earmold properly in the ear, the switches (including the use of the sound intensity control), the battery, the care of earmolds,

and others are presented to alleviate some of the difficulties some elderly residents may experience because of manual dexterity or memory problems. The staff of health care facilities can, further, aid the carryover of hearing aid orientation for recently fitted residents, if they are familiar with the component parts and their use.

5. Hearing aid troubleshooting procedures also are stressed and include:

 a. Knowledge of the causes of acoustic feedback (squealing)

 b. Battery longevity and placement

 c. Checking for cerumen (ear wax) in earmolds or hearing aid tubing

 d. Procedures for cleaning earmolds

 e. Correct use of the telephone switch and other controls

 Instructions to the staff of the health care facility on the care of hearing aids can be invaluable. The staff should be instructed to check to see that hearing aids do not go into the shower, the laundry, or denture cups, and that the hearing aids do not accidently get tossed out with soiled tissue paper, or flushed.

 The nurse aide, for example, can reduce a patient's stresses involved in adjusting to hearing aids by having the knowledge required to conduct a quick check on hearing aids that a frustrated elderly resident feels are not working. A simple adjustment of battery placement or reminding the resident that the earmolds need cleaning can eliminate non-use of otherwise beneficial hearing aids. Because these adjustments and reminders may be necessary when the audiologist is not in the health care facility, this aspect of in-service is *extremely* important. Loss of a hearing aid and battery problems are two of the most frequently observed problems for health care facility residents who have impaired hearing.

6. The components of a hearing rehabilitation program are discussed so that administration and staff are aware of the

intricacies involved not only in the assessment of auditory function, but also in treatment sessions. These insights and a resulting staff that is knowledgeable of the role of the audiologist, permits an enhanced working relationship between audiologist and staff.

The role of the staff in carryover is also discussed. This includes the fact that the staff can be the vital catalyst in providing an enhanced climate for communication in the health care facility.

7. Importantly, discussing methods for effective communication with hearing-impaired older adults is a critical part of in-service training. The stresses that grow out of frustrated attempts at communication, both on the part of residents and staff, can stifle an otherwise pleasant living environment. The suggestions provided the staff include the Thirteen Commandments for Communicating with Hearing Impaired Older Adults (Table 7–1; Hull, 1980).

PROVISION OF HEARING REHABILITATION TREATMENT SERVICES IN THE HEALTH CARE FACILITY

The specific strategies for providing aural rehabilitation treatment services on behalf of older adult patients in the health care facility include the following:

1. Motivation of residents,

2. The communicative/listening environment of the health care facility,

3. The health state of individual residents,

4. Family involvement, and

5. Compounding visual problems.

TABLE 7–1. The Thirteen Commandments for Communicating with Hearing-Impaired Older Adults

- Speak at a slightly greater than normal intensity.

- Speak at your normal rate, but not too rapidly.

- Do not speak to the elderly person at a greater distance than 6 feet but no less than 3 feet.

- Concentrate light on the speaker's face for greater visibility of lip movements, facial expression, and gestures.

- Do not speak to the elderly person unless you are visible to him or her (e.g., not from another room while he or she is reading the newspaper or watching TV).

- Do not force the elderly person to listen to you when there is a great deal of environmental noise. That type of environment can be difficult for a younger, normally hearing person. It can, on the other hand, be defeating for the hearing-impaired elderly.

- Never, under any circumstances, speak directly into the person's ear. Not only can the person not make use of visual clues, but the speaker may be causing an already distorting auditory system to distort the speech signal further. In other words, clarity may be depressed as loudness is increased.

- If the elderly person does not appear to understand what is being said, rephrase the statement rather than simply repeating the misunderstood words. An otherwise frustrating situation can be avoided in that way.

- Do not overarticulate. Overarticulation not only distorts the sounds of speech, but also the speaker's face, thus making the use of visual clues more difficult.

- Arrange the room (living room or meeting room) where communication will take place so that no speaker or listener is more than 6 feet apart, and all are completely visible. Using this direct approach, communication for all parties involved will be enhanced.

- Include the elderly person in all discussions about him or her. Hearing-impaired persons sometimes feel quite vulnerable. This approach will help alleviate some of those feelings.

TABLE 7–1. *continued*

- In meetings or any group activity where there is a speaker presenting information (church meetings, civic organizations, etc.) make it mandatory that the speaker(s) use the public address system. One of the most frequent complaints among elderly persons is that they may enjoy attending meetings of various kinds, but all too often the speaker, for whatever reason, tries to avoid using a microphone. Many elderly persons do not desire to assert themselves by asking a speaker who has just said, "I am sure that you can all hear me if I do not use the microphone," to please use it. Most persons begin to avoid public or organizational meetings if they cannot hear what the speaker is saying. This point cannot be stressed enough.

- Above all, treat elderly persons as adults. They, of anyone, deserve that respect.

Source: Reproduced with permission by Hull (1980b). The thirteen commandments for talking to the hearing-impaired older person. *Journal of the American Speech-Language-Hearing Association, 22,* 427.

Motivation

Some audiologists prefer not to attempt to provide aural rehabilitation services on behalf of older persons who reside in health care facilities. They reason that many potential patients lack the motivation necessary to benefit from their services. As clinicians observe these persons, many of them have good reason for their lack of motivation. Clinicians can, however, blame themselves for not providing the motivation. Cohen (1990) has described a number of reasons for lack of motivation among many elderly persons. Those may include, among others, a lack of available finances to purchase assistive listening devices, the death of a spouse or friends, lack of efficient modes of transportation, children living a great distance away, and physical problems that may restrict mobility.

Reasons for Lack of Motivation

As clinicians view elderly residents of health care facilities, they observe other more dramatic effects that impact on this population's motivation to receive rehabilitation services. According to early writings in Atchley (1972), Smyer, Zarit, and Qualls (1990), and Ronch (2009), the most depressing aspect of placement in a health care facility (nursing home) is the move from a home where the person may have lived for many years to a strange and, to that person, a probable final residence. The events leading to placement in the health care facility were, in all probability, equally stressful, including, perhaps, the loss of a spouse, the loss of a home due to rezoning laws or lack of finances, severe enough illness to require constant nursing care, or slowly declining health simply because of advancing age. If the elderly resident has read the statistics on the longevity of residents of nursing homes, he or she will know that the probability of survival after the first month of placement is only about 73%. Furthermore, only about 20% ever leave health care facilities except for burial (Moss & Halamandaris, 1997).

The well elderly in the community may not experience the reasons for depression, nor are they experiencing that single dramatic change in their lives. The fear of the necessity for a move to a health care facility can, however, result in motivation to work toward preventing it.

For those who can benefit from aural rehabilitation services, efforts toward motivation should be made. If for no other reason than to enhance communication abilities with family and friends in the confined environment of the health care facility, to be able to enjoy watching television once again, or to participate more efficiently in social activities within the health care facility, motivation for receiving aural rehabilitation services should be given a high priority. It must be kept in mind, however, as discussed in Chapter 4, the hearing rehabilitation treatment program must be developed around the patients' prioritized needs for communication, and no others.

Treatment Environment

Discovering an area within the health care facility where hearing rehabilitation and other specialized services can be provided in a pleasant and least restrictive environment can be challenging. Most health care facilities do have an area that is, at least, a pleasant place to be. That area may be an activity room, a lounge that is *not* the main lounge or lobby area, a staff dining room, or other sections of the health care facility that are not considered by the residents as ones where, for example, people go when they are "not well." Other places to avoid include the infirmary and the chapel.

The only available space where frequent disturbances may not occur may be an esthetically undesirable space, such as the laundry room or the rear portion of the cafeteria. In that instance, modifications will be necessary. This is not always greeted with enthusiasm by health care facility administrators, particularly with the tight budgets faced by many. Such modifications for improvement of the therapy environment, however, may be necessary for the aural rehabilitation program to be effective to any degree.

Some remodeling of an otherwise drab room can be done inexpensively. Some wallpaper, a movable partition, some paint, and carpeting can do wonders for the environment. There are few health care facilities that do not have at least a small amount of money for such improvements. If an audiologist has some talent for painting and hanging drapes, then labor costs may be reduced. Even some of the health care facility residents may enjoy chipping in on the labor. A retired carpenter or painter who resides in the health care facility may find it a joy to lend an experienced hand. Women who can make curtains may enjoy reawakening that skill for the good of the "Hearing Room." If the health care facility agrees to hire professionals to do the remodeling work, then such innovations may not be necessary.

At the University of Northern Colorado Aural Rehabilitation Program for the Aging that began in the middle of 1970s (Hull

& Traynor, 1976) and still thrives, installation of sound-treated rooms and audiometers, including carpentry, electrical work, painting, and others were funded by the health care facilities involved. When one health care facility was being constructed, the corporate owner's plans included a sound-treated room as part of the initial construction in support of their hearing rehabilitation program. The room, furthermore, was to double as a staff lounge. That aspect, for obvious reasons, was not a satisfactory arrangement, and the staff later found other quarters for coffee and conversation.

Another health care facility remodeled a large linen closet, one remodeled a large vacant resident room, and yet another built walls for a new room for the audiology services that was previously unused except for storage. Interest level in the program varies from facility to facility, but the general commitment remains the same. Figure 7–2 illustrates a desirable room arrangement for the provision of aural rehabilitation services, including counseling, hearing aid orientation, and discussions of difficult communication situations that patients face, and their resolution.

The Health Status of Patients

As stated earlier, an audiologist must be realistic regarding an elderly patient's potential to respond to aural rehabilitation services. A terminally ill resident of a skilled nursing wing of a health care facility may possess impaired hearing, but not be able to respond to a complex system of diagnostic evaluation. It is not reasonable to ask that person to participate in a complex aural rehabilitation program that involved problem solving and assertiveness training. However, as the result of effective in-service, a knowledgeable staff may ease some of the frustrations the resident may be having by using effective strategies for communication. If the state of health of some individuals was the catalyst for placement in the health care facility, but those persons can, indeed, benefit from audiology services, additional considerations will be necessary. For example, accommodations

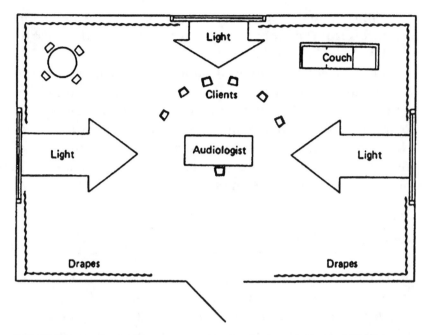

FIGURE 7–2. Desirable room arrangement for aural rehabilitation services in a health care facility.

for persons who are confined to a wheelchair are mandatory. Ramps into sound-treated testing booths, tables used in therapy that conform to the height of wheelchairs, and doors that permit maneuvering in and out of the rooms are necessary.

Attention Span

Many elderly persons cannot tolerate long periods of concentrated effort on any task. Audiometric evaluations in which attention to an almost inaudible pure tone is required, or aural rehabilitation sessions that instruct on more efficient means for communication, can become intolerable for some very elderly persons, even when the program is specifically designed around their needs. This is equally frustrating to some audiologists who have difficulty understanding the reason for the low attention/ tolerance span. The problem does exist, however and it must be accounted for.

It may be necessary to break audiologic evaluations into two or even three short periods, particularly if discussions regarding hearing aids are included. Hearing rehabilitation sessions should not last for more than 45 minutes. If patients appear to be less tolerant on a specific day, short breaks during which time something else is talked about may be necessary. An alert audiologist will realize when the "stretch breaks" are required.

Number of Patients for Group AR Sessions

The number of patients for optimal group interaction should not exceed six to eight. If at all possible, it is important to control admittance to specific groups to assure that hearing levels and levels of mental functioning among participants are as equal as possible. It can become frustrating for the group members, the audiologist, and the patient, if one patient has extreme difficulty communicating, or has difficulty participating in the group because of functional difficulties and demands the majority of attention. Out of necessity, the audiologist will tend to spend most of the group time attempting to facilitate that person's participation. The latter does not enhance positive and facilitatory group interaction. As the patients make progress in their communicative skill, the development of advanced classes may be warranted, depending on the needs of the patients.

Individual Versus Group Treatment

The more severely hearing impaired residents will require individual aural rehabilitation treatment. If a person progresses to the point that group involvement is possible, then he or she should be referred to that treatment setting. Some audiologists prefer to begin all patients' treatment on an individual basis so as to attend to any immediate needs they may have. And, some may never enter group treatment when their needs are met on an individual basis.

Acoustics and Lighting

Consideration of the acoustic and visual environment of an aural rehabilitation treatment facility is critical. At least initially, the environment should be a quiet one, free of undue reverberation, and with adequate lighting. Noting that older eyes generally will require as much as twice as much light as younger eyes, lighting is an important consideration.

Visual Aspects

Fluorescent lighting is not suggested for use with older patients. Both the hue of the light and the "flicker," even subliminal flicker, can cause visual difficulties, inattentiveness, and even seizures. Indirect and incandescent lighting is suggested, but glare from hard tables, floors, walls, and ceilings is to be avoided at all costs. Aging results in a thickening of the lens of the eye and a narrowing of the pupil aperture. Furthermore, the muscles of the eye do not function as quickly, so accommodations by older eyes for light changes are not as efficient.

Fozard (1990) and Woodruff (1975) wisely have advised that it takes almost twice the light energy to have the same effect on the older eye as the younger eye. In other words, the older eye is less responsive to light and cannot compensate for changes in light as quickly as it could when it was younger. It behooves the audiologist, therefore, to avoid moving from light to shadows as he or she is involved in aural rehabilitation treatment sessions.

Acoustic Needs

The suggested acoustic environment is one that consists of non-plush carpeted floors, textured walls, spackled acoustic tile ceilings or spackled dry wall, and chairs that at least have a padded seat and back. From this initial design, the audiologist can modify it to suit his or her own acoustic desires relative to aural rehabilitative tasks engaged in.

The room should not become so padded that it becomes anechoic, nor should it be too reverberant. A little reverberation gives sound "life." But, too much causes distortion of the acoustic aspects of speech. Unfavorable acoustics (reverberated speech) contributes greatly most to difficulties in speech understanding by older persons who have impaired hearing.

Time

The process involved in aural rehabilitation treatment can be fatiguing for both the patient and the audiologist. In providing services, particularly on behalf of the older adult patients, the factors of fatigue and alertness must be kept in mind. That includes remembering that most people function better at certain times of the day and that attention span and periods of maximum alertness are different as one becomes older.

When working with older adults, the period immediately following lunch, and anytime in the evening provides the least benefit. The inefficiency of those times is seen most dramatically among the confined or less active older person.

The time periods that are most advantageous for older adults are those toward the middle of the morning and perhaps 2 hours after lunch. The audiologist should be alert to the behaviors of his or her patients and change times as needed. It is generally best to ask the patient to suggest the time of day when he or she feels best.

The length of aural rehabilitation sessions must also be considered. This author has found that most alert, active older adults can work for at least 45 minutes to 1 hour, as long as periodic breaks are taken that include brief chats about things other than the treatment session. Many older patients will not be able to tolerate strenuous sessions for longer than 30 minutes. The alert audiologist will be able to judge the tolerance levels of his or her patients.

Family and Significant Others

Although the role of the family or other significant others in the aural rehabilitation process is discussed throughout this book, it is a critically important aspect to be presented as per the elderly adult who is confined to the health care facility. The discouraging component of this discussion, however, is that many family members of these persons either do not wish to become involved or live such a great distance away that they cannot be involved in any consistent manner. It is disheartening, not only on the part of the audiologist, but more so on the part of the elderly patient, to observe a family member who agreed to come to the health care facility to become involved in the aural rehabilitation process, who eventually dissolves the commitment. If such a possibility exists, it is generally better to not ask the family member to participate at all. A *genuine* commitment is necessary before such participation is initiated, mostly for the mental health of the elderly resident. The anguish felt by elderly persons, who eventually realize that their child or other family member apparently did not really desire to become involved, is heartbreaking.

If family involvement is possible, however, the enhanced awareness about the potential for communication by and with their family member can enhance family bonds. The importance of this involvement cannot be stressed enough.

Compounding Problems of Vision

The multiple handicaps of vision and hearing impairment are very real among elderly persons. Many of those with significant visual problems can be found within health care facilities, particularly if they have not been able to remain mobile and self-sufficient in their own homes.

For persons who have rehabilitative potential, the aural rehabilitation process revolves around working toward enhancement of auditory function, as visual clues may be of little advantage. The audiologist's efforts must be combined with those of a vision specialist who can work to assist a person in becoming more mobile, including correcting furniture arrangements in his or her room, safe use of cosmetics, and self-help skills. That team effort, along with the help of the Activity Director or Social Services staff of the health care facility can supplant the isolation that may otherwise face the elderly resident. The audiologist can play a vital role in providing input to the person's rehabilitation program.

SUMMARY

This chapter has presented considerations for the provision of services on behalf of persons who reside in health care facilities. It is stressed that, as with other patients, these persons' communication needs must be addressed as priorities. Even though they are residing within the confines of a health care facility, they are still individuals and, most importantly, they are individual adults with unique goals and concerns. The audiologist and other professionals who serve these people must be constantly aware of that fact. On the other hand, patients must be fully aware that they are involved in treatment, not simply another "activity" within the health care facility. They must be aware of the reasons for the communication problems they are experiencing, the steps that will be taken to help them, and the strategies involved. Only then will the services and the audiologist be accepted and meaningful.

References

Administration on Aging and the American Association of Retired Persons. *Profile of older Americans.* (2002). (Pub. No. PF3049, 1090). Washington, DC: Author.

Agrawal, Y., Platz, E., & Niparko, J. (2008). Prevalence of hearing loss and differences by demographic characteristics among U.S. adults. *Archives of Internal Medicine, 168*(14), 1522–1530.

Alpiner, J. G. (1963). Audiologic problems of the aged. *Geriatrics, 18,* 19–26.

Alpiner, J., & McCarthy, P. (Eds.). (1987). *Rehabilitative audiology: Children and adults* (Vol. 3). Baltimore, MD: Williams & Wilkins.

Atchley, R. C. (1972). *The social forces in later life.* Belmont, CA: Wadsworth.

Barnett, S., & Franks, P. (1999). Deafness and mortality: Analysis of linked data from National Health Interview Survey and National Death Index. *Public Health Report, 114*(4), 330–336.

Bayles, K. A., & Kaszniak, A. W. (1987). *Communication and cognition in normal aging and dementia.* Boston, MA: Little Brown.

Bergman, M. (1980). *Aging and the perception of speech.* Baltimore, MD: University Park Press.

Briner, W., & Willott, J. F. (1989). Ultrastructural features of neurons in the C57BL/6J mouse anteroventral cochlear nucleus: Young mice versus old mice with chronic presbycusis. *Neurobiology of Aging, 10,* 259–303.

Brody, H. (1955). Organization of the cerebral cortex. III. A study of aging in the human cerebral cortex. *Journal of Comparative Neurology, 102,* 511–556.

Caspary, D. M., Raza, A., Lawhorn-Armour, B. A., Pippin, J., & Arneric, S. P. (1990). Immunocytochemical and neurochemical evidence for age-related loss of GABA in the inferior colliculus: Implications for neural presbycusis. *Journal of Neuroscience, 10,* 2363–2372.

Castle, D. L. (1980). *Telephone training for the deaf.* Rochester, NY: National Technical Institute for the Deaf.

Centers for Disease Control and Prevention, & Agency for Toxic Substances and Disease Registry. (1999). *Simply put. Tips for creating easy-to-read print materials your audience will want to read and use.* Retrieved 10/2/2008, from http://www.cdc.gov/od/oc/simpput.pdf.

Cohen, G. D. (1990). Psychopathology and mental health in the mature and elderly adult. In J. E. Birren & K. W. Schaie (Eds.), *Handbook of the psychology of aging* (pp. 642–667). New York, NY: Academic Press.

Colton, J. (1977). Student participation in aural rehabilitation programs. *Journal of the Academy of Rehabilitative Audiology, 10,* 31–35.

Colton, J., & O'Neill, J. (1976). A cooperative outreach program for the elderly. *Journal of the Academy of Rehabilitative Audiology, 9,* 38–41.

Compton, C. L. (1989). Assistive devices. *Seminars in Hearing, 10,* 66–77.

Compton, C. L. (1993). Assistive technology for deaf and hard-of-hearing people. In J. G. Alpiner & P. A. McCarthy (Eds.), *Rehabilitative audiology: Children and adults* (2nd ed., pp. 440–468). Baltimore, MD: Williams & Wilkins.

Congdon, N., O'Colmain, B., Klaver, C., Klein, R., Munoz, B., Friedman, D. . . . Mitchell, P. (2004). Causes and prevalence of visual impairment among adults in the United States. *Archives of Ophthalmology, 122*(4), 477–485.

Dillon, H., James, A., & Ginis, J. (1997). The Client Oriented Scale of Improvement (COSI) and its relationship to several other measures of benefit and satisfaction provided by hearing aids. *Journal of the American Academy of Audiology, 8,* 27–43.

DiPietro, L., Williams, P., & Kaplan, H. (1984). *Alerting and communication devices for hearing impaired people: What's available now.* Washington, DC: National Information Center on Deafness, Gallaudet University.

Downs, M. (1970). *You and your hearing aid.* Unpublished manual. Denver, CO: University of Colorado Medical Center, Department of Otolaryngology, Division of Audiology.

Ebert, D. A., & Heckerling, P. S. (1995). Communication with deaf patients: Knowledge, beliefs, and practices of physicians. *Journal of the American Medical Association, 273*(3), 227–229.

Erber, N. P. (1985). *Telephone communication and hearing impairment.* San Diego, CA: College-Hill Press.

Erdmann, S. A. (1993). Counseling hearing-impaired adults. In J. G. Alpiner & P. A. McCarthy (Eds.), *Rehabilitative audiology: Children and adults* (2nd ed., pp. 374–413). Baltimore, MD: Williams & Wilkins.

Feeney, M. P., & Sanford C. A. (2004). Age effects in the human middle ear: Wideband acoustical measures. *Journal of the Acoustical Society of America, 116*(6), 3546–3558.

Fozard, J. (1990). Vision and hearing in aging. In J. E. Birren & K. W. Schaie (Eds.), *Handbook of the psychology of aging* (pp. 329–342). New York, NY: Academic Press.

Gaitz, C., & Warshaw, M. S. (1964). Obstacles encountered in correcting hearing loss in the elderly. *Geriatrics, 19*, 83–86.

Gatehouse, S. (1999). Glasgow Hearing Aid Benefit Profile: Derivation and validation of a client-centered outcome measure for hearing-aid services. *Journal of the American Academy of Audiology, 10*, 80–103.

Gates, G. A., Cobb, J. L., D'Agostino, R. B., & Wolf, P. A. (1993). The relation of hearing in the elderly to the presence of cardiovascular disease and cardiovascular risk factors. *Archives of Otolaryngology-Head and Neck Surgery, 119*(2), 156–161.

Gates, G. A., Couropmitree, N. N., & Myers R. H. (1999). Genetic associations in age-related hearing thresholds. *Archives of Otolaryngology-Head and Neck Surgery, 125*, 654–659.

Gatz, M., Bengtson, V. L., & Blum, M. J. (1990). Caregiving families. In J. E. Birren & K. W. Schaie (Eds.), *Handbook of the psychology of aging* (pp. 886–914). New York, NY: Academic Press.

Giolas, T. G. (1994). Aural rehabilitation of adults with hearing impairment. In J. Katz (Ed.), *Handbook of clinical audiology* (pp. 776–792). Baltimore, MD: Williams & Wilkins.

Glorig, A., & Davis, H. (1961). Age, noise, and hearing loss. *Annals of Otology, Rhinology, and Laryngology, 70*, 556–571.

Gordon-Salant, S., & Fitzgibbons, P. (2001). Source of age-related recognition difficulty for time-compressed speech. *Journal of Speech, Language and Hearing Research, 44*, 709–719.

Grady, C. L., & Craik, F. I. M. (2000). Changes in memory processing with age. *Current Opinion in Neurobiology, 10*, 224–231.

Grossman, B. (1955). Hard of hearing persons in a home for the aged. *Hearing News, 23*, 11–20.

Hardick, E. J. (1977). Aural rehabilitation programs for the aged can be successful. *Journal of the Academy of Rehabilitative Audiology, 10*, 51–66.

Health Care Financing Administration. (2004). *Incidence of health care facility placement in the U.S. Personal communication.* Washington, DC: Public Health Service.

Hellstrom, L. I., & Schmiedt, R. A. (1990). Compound action potential input/output functions in young and quiet-aged gerbils. *Hearing Research, 50*, 163–174.

Hellstrom, L. I., & Schmiedt, R. A. (1996). Measures of tuning and suppression in single-fiber and whole-nerve responses in young and quiet-aged gerbils. *Journal of the Acoustical Society of America, 100*, 3275–3285.

Helzner, E., Cauley, J., Pratt, S., Wisniewski, S., Zmuda, J., Talbott, E. O., . . . Newman, A. B. (2005). Race and sex differences in age-related hearing loss: The Health, Aging and Body Composition Study. *Journal of the American Geriatric Society, 53*(12), 2119–2127.

Hetu, R., Jones, L., & Getty, L. (1993). The impact of acquired hearing impairment on intimate relationships: Implications for rehabilitation. *Audiology, 32*, 363–381.

Hull, R. H. (1976). A linguistic approach to the teaching of speechreading: Theoretical and practical concepts. *Journal of the Academy of Rehabilitative Audiology, 9*, 14–19.

Hull, R. H. (1977). *Hearing impairment among aging persons*. Lincoln, NE: Cliff Notes.

Hull, R. H. (1980). Aural rehabilitation for the elderly. In R. L. Schow & M. A. Nerbonne (Eds.), *Introduction to aural rehabilitation* (pp. 311–348). Baltimore, MD: University Park Press.

Hull, R. H. (1980a). The thirteen commandments for talking to the hearing-impaired older person. *Journal of the American Speech and Hearing Association, 22*, 427.

Hull, R. H. (1982). *Rehabilitative audiology*. New York, NY: Grune & Stratton.

Hull, R. H. (1988). *Hearing in aging*. Presentation before the national invitational conference on Geriatric Rehabilitation. Department of Health and Human Services, PHS, Washington, DC.

Hull, R. H. (1989, November). *The use of interactive laser/video technology for training in visual synthesis and closure with hearing impaired elderly clients*. Presentation before the annual convention of the American Speech-Language-Hearing Association, St. Louis, MO.

Hull, R. H. (1992). Techniques for aural rehabilitation with elderly clients. In R. H. Hull (Ed.), *Aural rehabilitation: Serving children and adults* (pp. 278–292). San Diego, CA: Singular Publishing Group.

Hull, R. H. (1993). *Incidence of hearing loss in a nursing home population*. Unpublished study. Wichita State University, Wichita, KS.

Hull, R. H. (1997a). *Hearing in aging*. San Diego, CA: Singular Publishing Group.

Hull, R. H. (1997b). Techniques for aural rehabilitation treatment for older adults who are hearing impaired. In R. H. Hull (Ed.), *Aural rehabilitation: Serving children and adults* (pp. 367–393). San Diego, CA: Singular Publishing Group.

Hull, R. H. (1998). *Hearing in aging*. San Diego, CA: Singular Publishing Group.

Hull, R. H. (2001a). Aural rehabilitation for older adults with impaired hearing. In R. H. Hull (Ed.), *Aural rehabilitation: Serving children and adults* (pp. 393–424). San Diego, CA: Singular Publishing Group.

Hull, R. H. (2001b). Consideration for the use and orientation to hearing aids for older adults. In R. H. Hull (Ed.), *Aural rehabilitation: Serving children and adults* (pp. 373–392). San Diego, CA: Singular Publishing Group.

Hull, R. H. (2001c). Techniques of aural rehabilitation for older adults with impaired hearing. In R. H. Hull (Ed.), *Aural rehabilitation: Serving children and adults* (pp. 377–410). San Diego, CA: Plural Publishing.

Hull, R. H. (2006, November). *Addressing central auditory processing in aural rehabilitation for older adults*. Presentation at the annual convention of the American Speech-Language-Hearing Association, Miami, FL.

Hull, R. H. (2007). Fifteen principles of consumer-oriented audiologic/ aural rehabilitation. *ASHA Leader, 12*, 6–7.

Hull, R. H. (2009). *Introduction to aural rehabilitation*. San Diego, CA: Plural Publishing.

Hull, R. H. (2011). A brief treatise on the service of aural rehabilitation. *Hearing Journal, 64*, 14–16, 18.

Hull, R. H., & Traynor, R. (1976). A community-wide program in geriatric aural rehabilitation. *Journal of the American Speech-Language-Hearing Association, 14*, 33–34.

Humes, L. E. (2008). Aging and speech communication. *ASHA Leader, 13*, 10–13.

Ignatavicius, D. D., & Bayne, M. V. (1995). *Medical-surgical nursing*. Philadelphia, PA: W. B. Saunders.

Jerger, J. (1972). Audiological findings in aging. *Advances in Otorhinolaryngology, 20*, 115–124.

Jerger, J., & Chmiel, R. (1997). Factor analytic structure of auditory impairment in elderly persons. *Journal of the American Academy of Audiology, 7*, 269–276.

Kannapell, B., & Adams, P. (1984). *An orientation to deafness: A handbook and resource guide* (pp. 1–11). Washington, DC: Gallaudet University Press.

Kaplan, H. (1987). Assistive devices. In H. G. Mueller & V. C. Geoffrey (Eds.), *Communication disorders in aging* (pp. 464–493). Washington, DC: Gallaudet University Press.

Kaplan, H., Bally, S. J., & Brandt, F. D. (1990). *Communication skill scale.* Washington, DC: Gallaudet University.

Kaplan, H., Bally, S. J., & Garretson, C. (1987). *Speechreading: A way to improve understanding* (pp. 18–80). Washington, DC: Gallaudet University Press.

Kaplan, H. (2001). Counseling adults who are hearing impaired. In R. H. Hull (Ed.), *Aural rehabilitation* (pp. 207–226). San Diego, CA: Plural Publishing.

Kasten, R. N. (1981). The impact of aging on auditory perception. In R. H. Hull (Ed.), *The communicatively disordered elderly* (pp. 33–51). New York, NY: Thieme-Stratton.

Keithley, E. M., & Feldman, M. L. (1979). Spiral ganglion cell counts in an age-graded series of rat cochleas. *Journal of Comparative Neurology, 188,* 429–442.

Kirikae, I., Sato, T., & Shitara, T. (1964). Study of hearing in advanced age. *Laryngoscope, 74,* 205–221.

Kochkin, S. (2005). MarkeTrak VII: Hearing loss population tops 31 million people. *Hearing Review, 12*(7), 16–29.

Kochkin, S., & Rogin, C. (2000). Quantifying the obvious: The impact of hearing instruments on the quality of life. *Hearing Review, 7,* 6–34.

Kodman, F. (1967). *Techniques for counseling the hearing aid client. Maico audiological library series* (Vol. 8, Reports 23–25). Minneapolis, MN: Maico Hearing Instruments.

Lamb, S. H., Owens, E., & Schubert, E. D. (1983). The revised form of the Hearing Performance Inventory. *Ear and Hearing, 4,* 152–159.

Lee, F. S., Matthews, L. J., Dubno, J. R., & Mills, J. H. (2005). Longitudinal study of pure tone thresholds in older persons. *Ear and Hearing, 26,* 1–11.

Madden, D. (1985). Age-related slowing in the retrieval of information from long-term memory. *Journal of Gerontology, 40,* 208–210.

Marshall, L. (1981). Auditory processing in aging listeners. *Journal of Speech and Hearing Disorders, 46,* 226–240.

McCarthy, P. A., & Alpiner, J. G. (1978). The remediation process. In J. G. Alpiner (Ed.), *Handbook of adult rehabilitative audiology* (pp. 88–111). Baltimore, MD: Williams & Wilkins.

McCoy, S., Tun, P., Cox, L., Colangelo, M., Stewart, R., & Wingfield, A. (2005). Hearing loss and perceptual effort: Downstream effects on older adults' memory for speech. *Quarterly Journal of Experimental Psychology. A: Human Experimental Psychology, 58*(1), 22–33.

McCroskey, R. L., & Kasten, R. N. (1981). Assessment of central auditory processing. In R. Rupp & K. Stockdell (Eds.), *Speech protocols in audiology* (pp. 121–132). New York, NY: Grune & Stratton.

McLauchlin, R. (1992). Hearing aid orientation for hearing impaired adults. In R. H. Hull (Ed.), *Aural rehabilitation* (pp. 178–201). San Diego, CA: Singular Publishing Group.

Miller, M., & Ort, R. (1965). Hearing problems in a home for the aged. *Acta Oto-Laryngologica, 59,* 33–44.

Miller, W. E. (1976, November). *An investigation of the effectiveness of aural rehabilitation for nursing home residents.* Paper presented at the annual convention of the American Speech and Hearing Association, Houston, TX.

Mohr, P., Feldman, J., Dunbar, J. R., Niparko, J., Rittenhouse, R., & Skinner, M. (2000). The societal costs of severe to profound hearing loss in the United States. *International Journal of Technology Assessment in Health Care, 16*(4), 1120–1135.

Moss, F. E., & Halamandaris, F. E. (1997). *Too old, too sick, too bad: Nursing homes in America.* Germantown, MD: Aspen Systems.

O'Neill, J. J., & Oyer, H. J. (1981). *Visual communication for the hard of hearing.* Englewood Cliffs, NJ: Prentice-Hall.

Pichora-Fuller, M. K. (2006). Effects of age on auditory and cognitive processing: Implications for hearing aid fitting and audiologic rehabilitation. *Trends in Amplification, 10,* 29–59.

Plomp, R., & Mimpen, A. (1979). Speech-reception threshold for sentences as a function of age and noise level. *Journal of the Acoustical Society of America, 66*(5), 1333–1342.

Ramsdell, D. A. (1978). The psychology of the hard-of-hearing and the deafened adult. In H. Davis & S. R. Silverman (Eds.), *Hearing and deafness* (pp. 502–523). New York, NY: Holt, Rinehart, and Winston.

Rawool, V. W. (2007). The aging auditory system, Part 3: Slower processing, cognition, and speech recognition. *Hearing Review, 9,* 38–46.

Reuter-Lorenz, P. A. (2002). New visions of the aging mind and brain. *Trends in Cognitive Sciences, 6,* 394–400.

Reuter-Lorenz, P. A., Jonides, J., Smith, E., Hartley, A., Miller, A., Marchuetz, C., & Keoppe, R. (2000). Age differences in the frontal lateralization of verbal and spatial working memory revealed by PET. *Journal of Cognitive Neuroscience, 12,* 174–187.

Ronch, J. (2001). Who are these aging persons? In R. H. Hull (Ed.), *Aural rehabilitation: Serving children and adults* (pp. 295–310). San Diego, CA: Singular Publishing Group.

Ross, M. (1972). Hearing aid evaluation. In J. Katz (Ed.), *Handbook of clinical audiology* (pp. 482–513). Baltimore, MD: Williams & Wilkins.

Ross, M. (1982). *Hard-of-hearing children in regular schools.* Englewood Cliffs, NJ: Prentice-Hall.

Rupp, R. R., Higgins, J., & Maurer, J. F. (1977). A feasibility scale for predicting hearing aid use (FSPHAU) with other individuals. *Journal of the Academy of Rehabilitative Audiology, 10,* 81–104.

Sanders, D. A. (1982). *Aural rehabilitation.* Englewood Cliffs, NJ: Prentice-Hall.

Sanders, D. A. (1988). Hearing aid orientation and counseling. In M. C. Pollack (Ed.), *Amplification for the hearing impaired* (pp. 343–389). New York, NY: Grune & Stratton.

Sanders, D. A. (1993). *Management of hearing handicap.* Englewood Cliffs, NJ: Prentice-Hall.

Schmitt, J. F., & McCroskey, R. L. (1981). Sentence comprehension in elderly listeners: The factor rate. *Journal of Gerontology, 36,* 441–445.

Schow, R. L., & Nerbonne, M. A. (1980). Hearing levels in elderly nursing home residents. *Journal of Speech and Hearing Disorders, 45,* 124–132.

Schucknecht, H. F. (1974). *Pathology of the ear.* Cambridge, MA: Harvard University Press.

Schucknecht, H. F., & Gacek, M. R. (1993). Cochlear pathology in presbycusis. *Annals of Otology, Rhinology, Laryngology, 102*(1 Pt. 2), 1–16.

Schulte, B. A., Gratton, M. A., & Smythe, N. (1996). *Morphometric analysis of spiral ganglion neurons in young and old gerbils raised in quiet.* Paper presented at 19th Annual Midwinter Research meeting of the Association for Research in Otolaryngology, St. Petersburg, FL.

Smith, C. R., & Fay, T. H. (1977). A program of auditory rehabilitation for aged persons in a chronic disease hospital. *Journal of the American Speech and Hearing Association, 19,* 417–420.

Smyer, M. A., Zarit, S. H., & Qualls, S. H. (1990). Psychological intervention with the aging individual. In J. E. Birren & K. W. Schaie (Eds.), *Handbook of the psychology of aging* (pp. 375–394). New York, NY: Academic Press.

Stach, B. A. (1990). Central auditory processing disorders and amplification applications. *ASHA Reports, 19,* 150–156.

Stone, R., Cafferata, G. L., & Sangl, J. (1987). Caregivers of the frail elderly: A national profile. *Gerontologist, 36,* 616–626.

Suryadevara, A. C., Schulte, B. A., Schmiedt, R. A., & Slepecky, N. B. (2001). Auditory nerve gibers in young and aged gerbils: Morphometric correlations with endocochlear potential. *Hearing Research, 161,* 45–53.

Tarnowski, B., Schmiedt, R. A., Hellstrom, L. I., Lee, F., & Adams, J. (1991). Age-related changes in cochleas of Mongolian gerbils. *Hearing Research, 54,* 123–134.

Traynor, R., & Peterson, K. (1972). *Adjusting to your new hearing aid.* Unpublished manual. Greeley, CO.

Traynor, R. L. (1975). *A method of audiological assessment for the non-ambulatory geriatric patient.* Unpublished doctoral dissertation, University of Northern Colorado, Greeley, CO.

Tye-Murray, N. (1991). Repair strategy usage by hearing-impaired adults and changes following communication therapy. *Journal of Speech and Hearing Research, 34,* 921–928.

Tye-Murray, N. (1993). Aural rehabilitation and patient management. In R. S. Tyler (Ed.), *Cochlear implants: Audiological foundations.* San Diego, CA: Singular Publishing Group.

Tye-Murray, N., Purdy, S. C., & Woodworth, G. G. (1992). Reported use of communication strategies by SHHH members: Client, talker, and situational variables. *Journal of Speech and Hearing Research, 35,* 708–717.

US Census Bureau. (2008). *U.S. population projections.* Retrieved 9/25/2008, from http://www.census.gov/population/www/projections/files/nation/summary/np2008-t2.xls

Walden, B., Busacco, D., & Montgomery, A. (1993). Benefit from visual cues in auditory-visual speech recognition by middle-aged and elderly persons. *Journal of Speech and Hearing Research, 36*(2), 431–436.

Welsh, J., Welsh, L., & Healy, M. (1985). Central presbycusis. *Laryngoscope, 95,* 128–136.

Wingfield, A., McCoy, S., Peelle, J., Tun, A., & Cox, L. (2006). Effects of adult aging and hearing loss on comprehension of rapid speech varying in syntactic complexity. *Journal of the American Academy of Audiology, 17*(7), 487–497.

Woodruff, D. S. (1975). A physiological perspective of the psychology of aging. In D. S. Woodruff & J. E. Birren (Eds.), *Aging: Scientific perspectives and social issues* (pp. 179–198). New York, NY: Van Nostrand.

Working Group on Speech Understanding and Aging of the Committee on Hearing Bioacoustics and Biomechanics. (1988). Speech understanding and aging. *Journal of the Acoustical Society of America, 83,* 859–894.

Zafar, H. (1994). *Implications of frequency selectivity and temporal resolution for amplification in the elderly.* Unpublished doctoral dissertation, Wichita State University, Wichita, KS.

Zeng, F-G., Kong, Y-Y., Michalewski, H., & Starr A. (2005). Perceptual consequences of disrupted auditory nerve activity. *Journal of Neurophysiology, 93,* 3050–3063.

APPENDIX A

Suggestions for Coping in Difficult Listening Situations

■ Ask the speaker to speak in a good light and to face the listener, so that speechreading skills can be used.

■ Ask the speaker to speak clearly and naturally, but not to shout or exaggerate articulatory movements.

■ If you do not understand what a speaker is saying, ask the speaker to repeat or rephrase the statement.

■ If entering a group in the middle of a conversation, ask one person to sum up the gist of the conversation.

■ If someone is speaking at a distance, that person should be asked to stand closer.

■ If the speaker turns his or her head away, ask him or her to face you to permit optimal speechreading and listening.

■ If you are attempting to understand speech in the presence of noise, try to move yourself and the speaker away from the source of the noise.

■ When in a communication situation requiring exact information, such as asking directions or obtaining schedules for a trip, request that the speaker write the crucial information.

■ If the speaker is talking while eating, smoking, or chewing, request that he or she not do so, because it makes speechreading difficult.

■ A person who has a unilateral loss should be sure to keep the good ear facing the speaker at all times.

■ If possible, avoid rooms with poor acoustics. If meetings are held in such rooms, request that they be transferred to rooms with less reverberation.

■ If a speaker at a meeting cannot be heard, request that he or she use a microphone.

■ Arrive early for meetings, so that you can sit close to the speaker. Avoid taking a seat near a wall to minimize the possibility of reverberation. This is particularly important for those who use hearing aids.

■ If you are going to a movie or to the theater, read the reviews in advance to familiarize yourself with the plot.

■ In an extremely noisy situation, limit conversation to before the noise has started or after the noise has subsided. Normal hearing people do this all the time. For example, if a plane goes overhead and a conversation is going on, most people will halt their conversations and wait until the plane has passed.

Source: From Ackley, R. S. and Kaplan, H. (2009). Counseling adults who possess impaired hearing. In R. H. Hull, (Ed.), *Introduction to aural rehabilitation* (pp. 247–268). San Diego, CA: Plural Publishing. Reproduced with permission.

APPENDIX B

Books and Materials on Hearing Loss in Aging

The Consumer Handbook on Hearing Loss and
Hearing Aids: A Bridge to Healing
By Richard Carmen

Ideal for helping anyone who has a hearing deficiency to enjoy life to its fullest, this guide explores the causes and management of hearing loss and the corrective products and resources available. Readers will get professional advice on the choices of hearing devices as well as point-by-point explanations on types and care of aids and tips for extending the life of the mechanism. More than just a clinical aid, this guide also examines the anger, frustration, and denial often experienced by those with hearing loss and provides counsel to help deal with a variety of emotions. Also included is a resource section with contact information on national organizations that assist individuals with hearing impairments.

Hearing AIDS: The First 30 Days
By Jess Dancer

Taking the first step is always the hardest part of a journey. This easy-to-follow instructional handbook provides an abundance of information and advice for first time hearing aid users without being overwhelming. Written with care and understanding, this guide uses a combination of essays and exercises to help relieve anxiety and chart a course for success. A must read for patients, audiologists, and family members.

Consumer Handbook on Tinnitus
By Richard S. Tyler, PhD

Dr. Tyler has invited contributors from around the world to author a chapter in their specialty area of tinnitus. This is a one-of-a-kind book bound to make a difference to the hundreds of millions of people worldwide who experience persistent ringing or noises in their ears, millions of them completely disabled by it.

How Hearing Loss Impacts Relationships: Motivating Your Loved One
By Richard Carmen

Out of more than 28 million Americans with hearing loss, 80% of those people have not sought help for themselves. Among that 80%, many dismiss the extent of the problem or deny the existence of the problem. Most are resistant to seeking help, resulting in their loved ones enduring unnecessary strife and conflict.

This book is the first of its kind directed toward families. It explains how family members can manage the frustrations of a resistant loved one who won't seek treatment for hearing loss, and exposes the most common reasons behind the resistance. In addition to the fascinating insights into the psychology behind the resistance, it clarifies the family's role in shifting their loved one from "struggling to hear" to "hearing independence." This book will inspire readers to make the adjustments necessary to result in a higher quality of life for everyone. (Richard Carmen, AuD, [2005], 109 pages; soft cover)

The Consumer Handbook on Dizziness and Vertigo
By Dennis Poe

Educational and informative, *The Consumer Handbook on Dizziness and Vertigo* provides a comprehensive overview of this increasingly common condition. Loaded with practical information from the industry's top physicians, surgeons, and therapists, it reveals potential diagnoses, treatment options, surgical and nonsurgical alternatives, and methods of living with symptoms.

Overcoming Hearing Aid Fears—The Road to Better Hearing
By John M. Burkey

A hearing aid is a simple tool that can improve careers, relationships, and self-esteem. It can provide independence and security. Yet, only 20% of the nearly 30 million people with a hearing loss choose to use one despite the fact that technological advances have made hearing aids smaller and easier to use than those of the past.

This book can help readers take that first step. An audiologist himself, author John Burkey addresses common fears, concerns and misconceptions associated with hearing aids, providing practical information about styles, options, and costs. The book addresses the concerns people with hearing loss may experience, as well as help their family and friends understand why someone may resist getting a hearing aid. Audiologists will find this text an important educational tool in advising their own patients. ([2003], 175 pages; soft cover)

Hearing and Aging: Tactics for Intervention
By James F. Maurer and Ralph R. Rupp

This book describes the impact of aging and all that occurs with aging on hearing, and strategies for assisting older adults with impaired hearing.

Aging and the Auditory System: Anatomy, Physiology, and Psychophysics
By James F. Willott

Describes the aging auditory system, its anatomy, changes that occur in the physiology of the ear and its various parts as one ages, and how those changes impact on hearing.

Hearing Loss in the Elderly: Audiometric, Electrophysiological, and Histopathological Aspects
By Sava Soucek

Virtually everyone over the age of 70 suffers from a hearing loss. This is the conclusion reached in the study published here by two experts in audiology and ENT pathology. Deafness in old age is shown to be a specific condition caused by an innate degenerative change; specifically the loss of outer hair cells of the cochlea. Three lines of research are followed. The epidemiological line ties into audiometry for case detection. The electrophysiological line includes noninvasive techniques for detecting electrical responses from the cochlea. The histopathological line shows how special postmortem perfusion and slicing techniques are used to obtain satisfactory preparations. Most of the study is new and the results challenge current diffuse ideas and point to more rewarding areas of research.

The Official Patient's Sourcebook on Presbycusis: A Revised and Updated Directory for the Internet Age
By Icon Health Publications

Although it also gives information useful to doctors, caregivers and other health professionals, it tells patients where and how to look for information covering virtually all topics related to presbycusis (also sudden sensorineural hearing loss), from the essentials to the most advanced areas of research. The title of this book includes the word official. This reflects the fact that the sourcebook draws from public, academic, government, and peer-reviewed research. Selected readings from various agencies are reproduced to give you some of the latest official information available to date on presbycusis. Given patients' increasing sophistication in using the Internet, abundant references to reliable Internet-based resources are provided throughout this sourcebook. Where possible, guidance is provided on how to obtain free-of-charge, primary research results as well as more detailed information via the Internet. E-book and electronic versions of this sourcebook are fully interactive with each of the Internet sites mentioned (clicking on a hyperlink automatically opens your browser to the site indicated). Hard-copy users of this sourcebook can type Web addresses directly into their browsers to obtain access to the corresponding sites.

Quiet World: Living with Hearing Loss
By Professor David G. Myers

In this engaging and practical book, Myers, a social psychologist who has himself suffered gradual hearing loss, explores the problems faced by the hard of hearing at home and at work and provides information on the new technology and groundbreaking surgical procedures that are available to assist them. (6 illustrations)

Coping with Hearing Loss: Plain Talk for Adults About Losing Your Hearing
By Susan V. Rezen, and Carl D. Hausman

The reliable source for information on the emotional problems of hearing loss, doctors, types of hearing aids, and more including the latest technical and medical advances.

Hearing Aids
By Harvey Dillon

The complete, one-stop guide to hearing aids, covering everything you need to know to prescribe, select, fit, measure, and evaluate their performance. Dr. Dillon is a sought-after speaker and instructor throughout the world. Some of the benefits of this acclaimed text: *Comprehensive—From basic concepts of hearing loss, hearing aid software and hardware, to assessment guidelines and results-oriented counseling methods, the book covers it all! *Theoretically Sound—All findings explained in detail to clarify concepts, making the book ideal as a standard reference for clinicians as well as a core text in graduate courses. *Practical—Easy-to-use tips, tables, and procedures designed to be pinned to clinic walls for instant reference. *Accessible—Synopses, key paragraphs, and detailed materials help you progress from basic to highly sophisticated concepts easily. *Integrated and cross-referenced—Each cross-referenced chapter builds on previous chapters, with the flow and consistency of a single author. *Innovative—You will discover research results and procedures that have not yet appeared in the literature, giving you an important professional edge. Opinion leaders in the field have been uniformly enthusiastic:

> "The book is smashing . . . Should be a required reference for anyone who deals with hearing aids. All of the materials, including an outstanding chapter on pediatric amplification, are presented in a practical and immediately useful manner."
> —Jerry Northern, author and editor, HearX

> "Packed with concise, up-to-date, useful information concerning the selection and fitting of hearing aids. I'd highly recommend this text for graduate audiology students to anyone involved in hearing aid dispensing."—Gus Mueller, PhD, Adjunct Associate Professor, Vanderbilt University

Textbook of Hearing Aid Amplification: Technical and Clinical Considerations
By Robert E. Sandlin, PhD

This text provides the most current update of advances in hearing instrument technology and clinical practices associated with selection and fitting strategies. The text focuses on current practices related of the clinical assessment and decision-making processes. This is a valuable book for academic and clinical professionals involved in the selection and fitting of hearing aid devices for the acoustically impaired.

Strategies for Selecting and Verifying Hearing Aid Fittings
By Michael Valente (Editor)

This edition of a best-selling text is divided into four sections, organized to follow the sequence in which decisions are made regarding hearing aid fittings, and featuring new chapters on middle ear implants, hearing aid counseling, and infection control. Other chapters have been revised to reflect the latest developments in the field, such as: improving speech recognition with directional microphones; changing standards for measuring real-ear performance; and new prescriptive procedures for severe hearing loss. The text features contributions from internationally renowned experts in the field who share their extensive knowledge and clinical experience. It covers the six most common forms of hearing loss practitioners will encounter in their own practice — noise-induced, symmetrical, asymmetrical, unilateral, conductive, and severe hearing loss — with instructions on applying the newest technology to each hearing impaired group. Key features: Addresses the six most common types of hearing loss that comprise 90 to 95% of the situations audiologists encounter daily. Organized to follow the decision-making progress in selecting and verifying hearing aid fittings. Fully updated with state-of-the-art technology on implantable hearing aids, directional microphones, and more. A valuable glossary of terms at the end of the text — helpful for students and specialists alike. Together with its updated companion text, *Hearing Aids: Standards, Options, and Limitations*, this book forms the basis of a complete reference library on selecting, ordering, measuring, and verifying hearing aid fittings and performance

Hearing Loss Help: How You Can Help Someone with a Hearing Loss — And How They Can Help Themselves
By Alec Combs

This book describes strategies for helping individuals with impaired hearing, and helping them to help themselves.

Hearing Loss Help: For Yourself . . . for Someone
You Care About
By Alec Combs

Provides information that is complimentary to his sequel (above) on how to assist those who are close to us to cope with impaired hearing, and to function in difficult listening environments.

Overcoming Hearing Aid Fears: The Road to
Better Hearing
By John M. Burkey

A hearing aid is a simple tool to improve careers, relationships, and self-esteem, and to provide independence and security. Yet only 20% of people with hearing impairment choose to use one. *Overcoming Hearing Aid Fears* can help readers take that first step to a better life.

Hearing Better: Understanding Your Hearing and
Ear Care Options
By John M. Burkey, Franklin M. Rizer, MD, and Arnold G.
Schuring, MD

Shared authorship in writing this helpful book brings a wealth of understanding about the causes of hearing loss, how it may impact on those who possess it, and various options for reducing the handicap of hearing impairment.

Amplification for the Hearing-Impaired
By Michael C. Pollack (Editor)

This was a standard for many years on the topic of hearing aid evaluation and fitting primarily written for professionals in the field of audiology. It provides a wealth of information on hearing fitting options and strategies for evaluating and fitting hearing aids and other amplification systems on behalf of persons with impaired hearing.

Hearing Aid Handbook
By Jeffrey J. DiGiovanni

This unique desk reference on hearing aids gives unprecendented access to the major hearing aid manufacturers and their product lines, in a convenient "at-a-glance" format. Nine major manufacturer are profiled, with background information on each company including history, research and development, philanthropic activity, and warranty information. Following each profile is a comprehensive listing of that manufacturer's most current hearing aid products. This compendium of hearing aid information is essential for audiologists, hearing scientists, and anyone involved in the hearing aid industry.

Neurotransmission and Hearing Loss: Basic Science, Diagnosis and Management
By Charles I. Berlin (Editor)

Neurotransmission and Hearing Loss is the second book in the Kresge-Mimelsien award series, which emanates from a scientific symposium held annually to honor a scientist who has had a major impact on modern hearing research. In 1995, Dr. Robert Wenthold was chosen for his essential research in the biochemistry of synaptic transmission, the main theme of this scholarly work. The book covers both the basic science of neurotransmission and hearing loss and its clinical application, including Receptors in the Auditory Pathway, Transmitters in the Cochlea, Afferent Regulation of Cochlear Nucleus Neurons, Auditory Deprivation, and Genetic Disorders of the Auditory System. In the clinical segment, cochlear implants as a management tool for deafness are covered as well as audiological findings in autoimmune diseases, and with medical treatments for sensorineural loss and tinnitus. With contributions from the international and leading experts in the field, this book is an essential update on the literature in the field.

Modeling Sensorineural Hearing Loss
By Walt Jesteadt (Editor)

A recent study indicates that 20 million people in the United States have significant sensorineural hearing loss. Approximately 95 percent of those people have partial losses, with varying degrees of residual hearing. These percentages are similar in other developed countries. What changes in the function of the cochlea or inner ear cause such losses? What does the world sound like to the 19 million people with residual hearing? How should we transform sounds to correct for the hearing loss and maximize restoration of normal hearing? Answers to such questions require detailed models of the way that sounds are processed by the nervous system, both for listeners with normal hearing and for those with sensorineural hearing loss. This book contains chapters describing the work of 25 different research groups. A great deal of research in recent years has been aimed at obtaining a better physiological description of the altered processes that cause sensorineural hearing loss and a better understanding of transformations that occur in the perception of those sounds that are sufficiently intense that they can still be heard. Efforts to understand these changes in function have lead to a better understanding of normal function as well. This research has been based on rigorous mathematical models, computer simulations of mechanical and physiological processes, and signal processing simulations of the altered perceptual experience of listeners with sensorineural hearing loss. This book provides examples of all these approaches to modeling sensorineural hearing loss and a summary of the latest research in the field.

APPENDIX C

Selected Resources for Assisting Older Adults with Impaired Hearing

Starkey's Web site promotes their hearing aids, shows different places where disadvantaged older adults can go to apply for free hearing aid, and keeps up with hearing news.
http://www.starkeyhearingfoundation.org/

Oticon's Web site provides several articles on their hearing aids and hearing loss.
http://www.healthyhearing.com

Phonak's Web site is very detailed goes into the explanation of why we have hearing loss and shows how their products can help.
http://www.phonak.com/us/b2c/en/home.html

California Ear Institute's Web site is very detailed in what it has to offer adults in the form of hearing aids, implants and surgeries especially with new information on atresia repair and tinnitus.
http://www.californiaearinstitute.com/

Web Sites Geared Toward Adults

These Web sites are geared toward the aging adult who needs resources and help.

Center of Hearing and Communication is geared toward hearing aids, based in Florida and New York. Brief overview of hearing loss and tinnitus.
http://www.chchearing.org/

Better Hearing Web site gives very brief but well-detailed information on hearing loss, hearing aids, and other information people need to know about hearing.
http://www.betterhearing.org/

CDC (Centers for Disease Control) is a government site that has a great deal to offer in noise prevention and how it occurs.
http://www.cdc.gov/niosh/topics/noise/default.html

National Institute on Deafness Web site gives several well-detailed answers on pathologies for people who are searching for more information, ranging from auditory neuropathy to Waardenburg syndrome.
http://www.nidcd.nih.gov/health/hearing/

"Hear It" Web site comes in many different languages and has a great deal of information on hearing loss and what can damage hearing.
http://www.hear-it.org/

American Association of Retired Persons (http://www.AARP .org) has information on hearing loss and its link to symptoms of dementia. The reader is warned that information on this site is somewhat difficult to find and one must look in all of its links to find what is being searched for.
http://www.aarp.org/health/medical-research/info-02-2011/hearing_loss_linked_to_dementia.html

AARP and Hear USA Web site to help those who need info on how to obtain hearing aids
http://aarp.hearusa.com/

Mayo Clinic Web site gives very brief and detailed information on hearing loss.
http://www.mayoclinic.com/health/hearing-loss/DS00172

Very detailed Web site on all aspects of audiology, gives the user several answers to different questions, and has a great wealth of detail on several pathologies.
www.audiologyonline.com

Web site that gives very brief information on hearing loss and how to obtain help.
www.howsyourhearing.org/

Very good Web site from the United Kingdom provides a great deal of information from articles and information from around the world.
http://www.aud.org.uk/contents/contents.htm

Very detailed Web site of the American Speech-Language-Hearing Association that gives the public several options and information on hearing loss.
http://www.asha.org/

The American Tinnitus Association Web site gives a great deal of info on tinnitus and how to accept it and treat it.
http://www.ata.org/

Web site that gives very detailed information on inner ear disorders.
http://www.vestibular.org/

Index